Adverse Effects of T[illegible]n M[illegible]

MW01674368

by

P K ARIVAL

Copyright © [2023]

Title: Adverse Effects of Trace Metals on Male Infertility

Author's: P K Arival

All rights reserved. No part of this publication may be reproduced stored in a retrieval system, or transmitted in any form or by any means electronic, mechanical, photocopying, recording, or otherwise, without the prior written permission of the publisher or author, except in the case of brief quotations embodied in critical reviews and certain other non-commercial uses permitted by copyright law

This book was printed and published by [P K Arival in [2023]

ISBN: 9781805250623

For permission to reproduce any of the material in this book.

INDEX

LIST OF TABLES

LIST OF FIGURES

1.0 INTRODUCTION

A disease in the reproductive system of human, failure to get pregnant after the year or more of regular unprotected sexual practice is defined as infertility. Infertility is not only a disease but it's a condition with psychological, stress, economic and social pressure on child-bearing (Zegers-Hochschild *et al.*, 2009). It is obvious that it regular problem affecting not only young couples but also for older ones, and equally clear that it results in considerable distress for those couples affected. Few feelings faced by infertile couples like anger for no reason, high depression, and shame on themselves, isolation from family members, social pressure and embarrassment in front of fertile couples (Wright *et al.*, 1991). Varicocele factor responsible for male infertility is identified in 50% of these couples (AUA, 2012). Infertility in the male has been identified due to various environmental, biochemical and genetic factors, which includes lifestyle changes, hormonal imbalance, abnormal chromosomes, and problems in ejaculation, varicoceles, testicular failure and exposure to gonadotoxin. Since male infertility now becomes the worldwide health issues, it is necessary to evaluate and to provide treatment to reduce the prevalence of male infertility. Other options such as assisted reproductive techniques (ART) may also available to achieve pregnant. Nearly 8% of the male at reproductive stage need medical help for reproductive issues, of which, 1–10% of male not potential reproductive and 30% of them have a varicocele. A Multi-centric study conducted by WHO between 1982 and 1985 indicates 20% of infertility cases were due to male factors, 38% of female factors, 27% of both, and 15% could not be satisfactorily attributed to either partner (WHO, 1987).

1.1 International prevalence of infertility

Globally 40–50% of fertility problem are due to only male factors, which is affecting 10–15% of the reproductive age of couples (Rutstein and Shah, 2004). In developed and in developing countries the prevalence of male infertility is varying based on the resources for investigation and treatment are available. Around 60-80 million couples suffer from infertility every year in the world, of which 15–20 million from India (Mehrotra *et al.*, 2013). In the countries like the UK and USA, it is estimated that 6–10% of males have fertility problem (Ugwuja *et al.*, 2008). Studies conducted in Denmark evaluate that 15.7% of the male with poor semen quality (Schmidt *et al.*, 1995). Developing countries like Nigeria have 30% of male infertility rate (Larsen, 2000). Some of the regions in the world like South Asia, sub-Saharan Africa, the Middle East, North Africa, Central Eastern Europe and Central Asia have much higher male infertility rate (Nachtigall, 2006; Ombelet *et al.*, 2008a & b and Mascarenhas *et al.*, 2012b). In a study conducted in France during 1988–1989, the incidence of infertility amongst couples has been estimated to be 14% (Thonneau *et al.*, 1991). In the United States of America (USA), 10% to 20% of couples are estimated to be infertile (Jacobs, 1988). A new study conducted from the Hebrew University of Jerusalem shows that the sperm counts of those males from North America, Europe, Australia and New Zealand were declined about 50-60% from 1973–2011 (Levine *et al.*, 2017). A research study reported the prevalence of infertility in Pakistan is 21% of which 35% is contributed by the male factor (Zahid *et al.*, 2015). Recent report reveals that the male infertility rate at younger than age 30 years has also increased worldwide by 15% (Martin *et al.*, 2009) and then it shows the male infertility in worldwide, 59% in France, 36% in South Africa, Indonesia and Finland, 35% in Nigeria and some parts of sub-Saharan Africa including the Republic of Sudan and Cameroon, 26–32% in Kashmir Valley (India) and UK and 10% in USA (Thonneau *et al.*, 1991; Mehta *et al.*, 2006; Fisch and Goluboff, 1996; Okonofua *et al.*, 1997 and Schmidt *et al.*,1995).

1.2 National prevalence of infertility

The infertility rate in India has also increased gradually along with the population growth (Seshagiri, 2001). Based on the geographic; the prevalence of male infertility varies. However, according to a study by WHO, the incidence of infertility in India is not yet clear. It is estimated that approximately 13 to 19 million couples are infertile (Sharma *et al.*, 2005). As per the WHO, the overall prevalence of primary infertility ranges between 3.9% and 16.8% (Calverton, 2004) Also, the estimates of infertility vary widely among Indian states from 3.7% in Uttar Pradesh, Himachal Pradesh and Maharashtra, (Talwar *et al.*,1986) to 5% in Andhra Pradesh (Unisa, 1999) and 15% in Kashmir (Zargar *et al.*, 1997). In Kanyakumari district, the incidence of male infertility was found around 17% (Shamila and Sasikala, 2011). A study conducted to determine regional variation in the prevalence of azoospermia, oligozoospermia and mean sperm counts in male partners of infertile couples from different parts of India shows that it was a regional variation in the prevalence of azoospermia. The prevalence of azoospermia was extremely high in Kurnool and Jodhpur (38.3% and 37.4%, respectively). There was also a regional variation in the prevalence of oligozoospermia (51%) in Kurnool (Mehta *et al.*, 2006). Region wise distribution in India shows that North with high infertility when compared to south region (Dyson and Moore, 1983).

1.3 Etiology of male infertility

There are many factors responsible for male infertility such as auto immunological problem, abnormal endocrine function, abnormalities and infection in the genital tract, abnormal gene pattern, and changes in healthy lifestyle and exposure to gonadotoxic factors (Nieschlag, 2000). In addition to these factors idiopathic and unexplained male infertility (UMI) are also the main cause of male infertility. In men, many physiological activities like sperm production, sperm count and motility of sperm are strongly influenced by genetic factors (Katherine *et al.*, 2010). A mutation in cystic fibrosis transmembrane conductance regulator (CFTR) gene which causes cystic fibrosis (CF) is the most common abnormal gene functions. Congenital absence of the vas deferens (CAVD) is another cause of infertility in men with low semen level with acidic pH (Pauer *et al.*, 1997). Earlier study showed that patients with primitive testiculopathy produce a greater number of spermatozoa with aneuploidies compared to subjects with normal parameters of the seminal fluid, in spite of the presence of a normal karyotype (Calogero *et al.*, 2001). Y chromosome micro deletions are a frequent cause of infertility in males (Schlegel, 2004). Some genes located on the Y chromosome are suggested as candidates for the conditions like azoospermia and oligozoospermia (Ozdemir *et al.*, 2020). Development of male germ cell is always dependent on the function of endocrine glands like hypothalamus, pituitary and the testis (de Kretser, 1979). Hormones include FSH, LH and Testosterone are required for the proper production and maintenance of sperm production. Production of sperm and secretion of male sex hormones are the two main functions of the testis. These two functions are highly maintained by the pituitary gonadotropins, follicle-stimulating hormone (FSH) and luteinizing hormone (LH). Failure of hormone production results in abnormal function of testis leading to male infertility (Weinbauer and Nieschlag, 1995).

Table 1: The prevalence of causes of male infertility (Rowe *et al.*, 1993)

Infertility Causes	Prevalence (%)
Gonadotrophin deficiency	>0.1
Pituitary lesions	>0.1
Immotile clia syndrome	>0.1
Retrograde ejaculation	0.1
Partial obstruction to ejaculatory duct	0.1
Karyotype abnormalities	0.1
Latrogenic causes	0.5
Hyperprolactinaemia	0.6
Ejaculatory inadequacy	0.7
Idiopathic necrozoospermia	0.8
Obstructive azoospermia	0.9
Sexual inadequacy	1.3
Systemic diseases	1.4
Congenital abnormalities	1.7
Suspected immunological infertility	3.0
Isolated seminal plasma abnormalities	3.5
Idiopathic asthenozoospermia	3.9
Idiopathic teratozoospermia	5.9
Accessory gland infection	6.9

Table: 2 Nomenclature related to semen quality (WHO, 2010)

Aspermia	No semen during ejaculation.
Asthenozoospermia	Percentage of motile sperm below the lower reference limit.
Asthenoteratozoospermia	Percentage of motile sperm and normal sperm morphology below the lower reference limit.
Azoospermia	Total absence of sperm in the ejaculated semen.
Cryptozoospermia	Absence of sperm in fresh ejaculated semen but present in centrifuged pellet.
Haemospermia	Presence of RBC in the semen.
Leukospermia	Presence of leukocytes in the semen higher than threshold value.
Necrozoospermia	Low percentage of live sperm and high percentage of dead sperm in the semen.
Normozoospermia	Total count of sperm with normal motility and no morphology changes, equal or above the lower reference limit.
Oligoasthenozoospermia	Total count and percentage of motile sperm below the lower reference limit.
Oligoasthenoteratozoospermia	Total count, percentage of motility and normal morphology of sperm below the lower reference limit.
Oligoteratozoospermia	Total count and normal morphology of sperm below the lower reference limit.
Oligozoospermia	Total count of sperm below the lower reference limit.
Teratozoospermia	Percentage of normal morphological sperm below the lower reference limit.

1.3.1 Idiopathic impairment of the semen quality

The major cause of impaired semen parameters in the reported cases of male infertility is not clear. The absence of sperm in the testis (azoospermia) or sperm density <15 million per mL (oligozoospermia) may have a strong relationship with the soft tissues in the testis, abnormal hormonal secretion, and histological changes in the seminiferous tubules such as absence or the low number of male gametes. Sperm with poor motility less than 32% (asthenozoospermia) or total absence of motility may cause by morphology abnormalities (Opsahl *et al.*, 2000). Structural changes in sperm (teratozoospermia) may reflect on immaturities and low functional integrity of sperm (Paulson *et al.*, 1991). Ten percent of reported male infertility cases were diagnoses azoospermia. There are many causes of azoospermia-like testicular insufficiency, the barrier in the genital tract (Hendry *et al.*, 1994). A few years ago men with azoospermia were reported as infertile and the doctor advised to get donor sperm for conceiving but due to the development in the medical technologies the andrologist may extract the sperm from the epididymis, thus the azoospermia men get a child through ART procedure. To confirm the diagnose the azoospermia, the semen analysis should be examined twice in two weeks interval according to WHO guidelines (WHO, 2010). Oligozoospermia has divided into two types based on the sperm count per milliliter. Those who have sperm count less than 10×10^6 is called permanent oligozoospermia and those who have sperm count more than 10×10^6 is called periodic oligozoospermia. A clinical research study conducted in 1864 patients reported that the overall prevalence of oligozoospermia was observed as 16.6%. Among that 12.3% was permanent and 4.3% was periodic oligozoospermia respectively. Different sperm count ranges were statistically set by many authors to define oligozoospermia (Van Zyl, 1976). Definition of the oligozoospermia with the sperm count less than 60×10^6/mL (Tyler and Singher, 1956), 40×10^6/mL (William, 1964), 20×10^6/mL (MacLeod and Gold, 1951b), 10×10^6/mL (Santamauro *et al.*, 1972). Percentage of morphologically normal sperm observed lesser than the lower reference limit is defined as teratozoospermia (Ombelet *et al.*, 1995). Changes in sperm morphology have been associated with higher reactive oxygen species (ROS) leads the damage of sperm and cause infertility (Agarwal *et al.*, 2014). The success rate of IVF and embryo transfer was correlated with teratozoospermia. It is observed that low IVF success rate due to poor fertilization capacity in participants with teratozoospermia (Terriou *et al.*, 1997). A research study suggests that there is no correlation between sperm morphology and ICSI outcomes

(Colturato *et al.*, 2008). Study shows that sperm morphology is one of the markers to analysis the fertilization rate and embryo development in ART cycles (Hammoud *et al.,* 2008).

1.3.2 Varicocele

Abnormal dilation of veins of pampiniform plexus that drains the testis is called varicocele. Recent research work has found that due to varicocele many changes happen at the molecular level in the reproductive system which includes increased oxidative stress, higher testicular temperature, hypoxia and stasis. The temperature of the scrotum is maintaining a few degrees below when compared to body temperature to maintain the optimal sperm production and function (Dahl and Herrick, 1959). Due to the high blood flow of testicular veins, the temperature of the scrotum has raised and decreased the sperm quality lead to male infertility (Unsal *et al.*, 2007). Turkyilmaz *et al.*, (2004), conducted a study to compare the adolescent with and without varicoceles, Nitric oxide concentration in testicular veins was observed higher when compared to the control group. Esteves *et al.*, (2010) conducted a research study in a 242 infertile male who underwent ICSI with and without varicocele. The study results show that a higher birth rate was observed in men who underwent varicocele surgery before ICSI as compare to men who underwent ICSI with varicocele. Haans *et al.*, (1991) conducted the study to conclude that varicocele causes either failure or increase the weight of the testis. It is concluded that varicocele can cause the damage to the tissues of the testis, which leads to reducing the testis weight. Many other studies also supported that varicocele have strong relationship with semen parameters like sperm count, motility, volume, pH and success rate in ART techniques (Lund *et al.*, 1999 and Naughton *et al.*, 2001).

1.3.3 Genetic abnormalities

Changes in the chromosomes or mutation in the gene can directly affect the sperm production and the barrier in the sperm flow track that lead to male infertility. Males with multiple karyotype abnormalities also increase the production of aneuploid sperm. The severity of male infertility based on the proportion of the chromosomal abnormalities and pregnancy loss, embryo developmental disorder may cause due to chromosomal aneuploidy (Hassold *et al.*, 2001). Many studies reviewed the process of aneuploidy and study result concluded that chromosomal abnormalities lead to disturbance in meiotic cell division in male gametes, separation of sperm DNA chromatids and mitotic cell division in the embryo after fertilization of sperm with abnormal DNA (Gabriel *et al.*, 2011 and Kuliev *et al.*, 2011).

Many studies examine the level of sperm aneuploidy in both fertile and infertile male using FISH technique. It is evident from these studies that both fertile and infertile participants have aneuploidy sperm in their ejaculate semen. The level of aneuploidy in infertile men was reported at about 3-5% and it also states that the level of aneuploidy was found higher proportion in infertile men when compared to fertile men. The severity of chromosomal abnormalities was observed in all types of male infertility like asthenozoospermia (poor motility), oligozoospermia (low concentration), teratozoospermia (poor morphology) and azoospermia (absence of sperm) (Shi and Martin, 2001). A deletion in Y chromosomes is one of the most genetic causes of male infertility. There are 3 types of azoospermia factors have identified in the long arm of the Y chromosome. Deletions in such region cause multifunctional defects in sperm production and the prevalence of male infertility are based on the number of deletions (Simoni, 2001).

1.3.4 Male accessory gland infection

A wide range of harmful microorganisms was observed in the male urogenital tract which is associated with poor semen quality especially motility, function and DNA integrity. Identification of contaminating microorganism in prostate secretion was examined by culture test and antibiotics are selected based on the microorganism nature. Many *in vitro* studies have reported that presence of *E.coli* on semen has directly affected the sperm function (Diemer *et al.*, 1996; Huwe *et al.*, 1998 and Diemer *et al.*, 2003b). A normal spermatozoon incubated with *E.coli* culture was observed apoptosis in sperm after the incubation period. Thus the result of these studies suggests that *E.coli* contamination directly modify the ejaculate sperm function without interfering the sperm molecular mechanism. Similarly like *E.coli and* other microorganism contamination like *Neisseria gonorrhoeae* (Liu *et al.*, 2002 and Binnicker *et al.*, 2003), *Chlamydia trachomatis* (Gallegos *et al.*, 2008 and Kokab *et al.*, 2010), *Ureaplasma urealyticum* (Wang *et al.*, 2006 and Zheng *et al.*, 2008), *Mycoplasma hominis* (Gallegos *et al.*, 2008 and Gdoura *et al.*, 2008), *Candida albicans* (Tian *et al.*, 2007 and Rennemeier *et al.*, 2009), *Trichomonas vaginalis* (Kranjcic-Zec *et al.*, 2004 and Benchimol *et al.*, 2008), Hepatitis B and C viruses (Lorusso *et al.*, 2010) and Human immunodeficiency virus type 1 (Nicopoullos *et al.*, 2004 and Umapathy, 2005) have negative correlation with poor semen quality lead to male infertility.

1.3.5 Isolated seminal plasma abnormalities

Human seminal plasma is a clear liquid in nature but due to the presence of higher level WBC and mucous streaks, it becomes cloudy. Due to lower prostate secretion, seminal plasma liquefaction is poor (Elzanaty *et al.*, 2002 & 2004). These changes in seminal plasma may change the normal sperm number, motility and morphology leads to poor transport in cervical mucus and decrease the chance of conception. Evidence from the research study suggesting that abnormal seminal plasma may influence the sperm function (Carpino *et al.*, 1994), chromatin stability (Gonzales and Sanchez, 1994) and lower level of zinc and calcium (Malm *et al.*, 2000). The abnormal epididymal function may have a negative association with the decreased antioxidant function of the seminal plasma leads to imbalance oxidative stress and antioxidant protection compound (Koca *et al.*, 2003). Participants with male accessory gland infection, inflammation of seminal vesicle and varicocele or hypoandrogenism were reported to have abnormal seminal plasma. A huge number of tissues specific proteins in the seminal plasma which has specific functions in the male reproductive system. Due to reproductive disorders, the proteins in the seminal plasma get altered and become functionally defects. These proteins are used as biomarkers to access male infertility by mass spectrometry. These functional proteins can appear earlier in seminal plasma than blood; this facilitates the early detection of diagnosis of prostate cancer (Drabovich *et al.*, 2014). Another seminal biomarker which presents in epididymal fluid and plasma are hexosaminidase (Hex), which is the most active glycoside used to diagnose azoospermia. Hex activity was significantly decreased in azoospermic semen sample due to a lower concentration of respective enzymes. Hex activities have a positive correlation with motility in asthenozoospermic male and negatively correlate with azoospermic males (Menendez-Helman *et al.*, 2015). A study conducted to analyze the immunomodulatory potential of seminal plasma of men with and without fertility problem. The results show that there is no significant differences were observed in immunomodulatory potential of seminal plasma of both fertile and infertile groups (Von Wolff *et al.*, 2007). Role of malondialdehyde and ascorbic acid in male fertility was studied in normozoospermia, oligoasthenoteratozoospermia, asthenoteratozoospermia and azoospermia. The result shows that malondialdehyde was observed lower in normal group than in abnormal. Ascorbic acid was observed higher level in normal when compared to the abnormal group. Malondialdehyde was negatively correlated and ascorbic acid was positively correlated with semen parameters like count, motility and morphology (Das *et al.*, 2009).

1.3.6 Immunological infertility

Infertility caused by immune attacks on the tissues involved in the reproduction leads to male infertility is called immunological infertility. Unlike other cells in the organism, the sperm cells start producing only at the time of reproductive age. During that age, the immune system of the organism well develops and produce various antibodies against the antigen. The body will detect sperm as antigen due to new production in the body. Autoimmune infertility in man caused by the immune system produces antibodies against own sperm cells leads to disturbance in sperm production and changes in morphology and unable to fertilize an egg. It was observed that participants who undergone vasectomy surgery may have the high risk of autoimmune infertility. After vasectomy surgery, there no longer release of sperm in the body. The immune system of the body produces antibodies (Anti-sperm antibodies) to clear and engulf the unreleased sperm (Hassoun *et al.*, 1991). A study was conducted to examine the immune suppression treatment in infertile men who were diagnosed has immunological infertile. The participants were taken 96 mg per day methylprednisolone for 7 days. The results show that there is a drastic decrease in Acid soluble glycoproteins (ASP) level in blood and improved in pregnancy rate after successful immunosuppression treatment (Shulman *et al.*, 1978). ASA has a wide range of impact on male infertility which includes decreasing the sperm production leads to oligozoospermia and azoospermia, binding of antibodies in sperm leads to disturbance in sperm transport in male reproductive tract, agglutination of ejaculated semen and antibodies on sperm surface receptors may block the sperm-ovum interaction (Heidenreich *et al.*, 1994). One year of methylprednisolone treatment of immunologic infertility in the male was observed and the results show that increased the fertility rate (Shulman JF and Shulman S, 1982).

1.3.7 Congenital abnormalities and male infertility

Congenital abnormalities of the male are the structural defect in the genital tract right from the birth. It very hard to diagnose these defects at the younger age and some of them can be diagnosed after the development of symptoms at reproductive age. Congenital abnormalities in male basically happen during the early development of the fetus in the mother womb. This defect might change the functional and structural of the genital tract which may cause by chromosome abnormalities, harmful substance exposure of the fetus. One of the most common congenital abnormalities in boys is undescended testes. In this case, the testis fails to come down to the scrotum and remain in the pelvic area and become dysfunctional. Thus the production and function of sperm was affected leads to male infertility and have a high risk of testicular cancer (Coffee *et al.*, 2009). The prevalence of cryptorchidism in the full-term baby was about 1–3% and 30% in premature babies (Kolon *et al.*, 2004). Many research studies conducted to conclude that there is a negative correlation between cryptorchidism and male infertility (Trussel and Lee, 2004). Another congenital anomaly is Hypospadias were there is an arrest in normal development of urethra and penis. The phenotype changes range from a mild percentage (distal glandular meatus) to a high percentage (Ambiguous Genitalia) (Warren, 2016). Parental abnormalities like low sperm count, abnormal morphology leads to hypospadias in offspring (Fritz and Czeizel, 1996). As these offspring reach the reproductive age there is a sexual function issue.

1.3.8 Systemic diseases and male infertility

Many systemic diseases can have negative feedback on poor semen quality leads to male infertility. Many results confirmed that diseases like renal failure (Bundschu *et al.*, 1976), febrile illness (Carlsen *et al.*, 2003), liver cirrhosis (Castilla-Cortazar *et al.*, 2004), hyperparathyroidism (Chou *et al.*, 2003), cancer (Deane *et al.*, 2004), influenza and high fever (Evenson *et al.*, 2000), HIV (Sauer, 2005), spinal cord injury (Padron *et al.*, 1997), diabetes mellitus (Sexton and Jarow, 1997), have strong negative impact on male infertility. The study was conducted to examine the association between periodontal status and idiopathic male infertility and results show that there is no significant association between the poor periodontal status and male infertility (Pasztor *et al.*, 2016). A case-control study conducted in untreated psoriasis subject to examine the association of male infertility and study data concludes that there is a negative correlation between psoriasis and poor semen quality (Caldarola *et al.*, 2017). Diabetes may change the modification genes of the sperm during spermatogenesis and these changes can be inherited to next generation through sperm which turns high risk of diabetes in the progeny (Ding *et al.*, 2015). The wide range of cancer medicines, chemotherapy, radiotherapy, and surgery have shown strong effects on poor semen quality like sperm count, density, morphology, ejaculate volume etc (Meirow and Schenker, 1995).

1.4 Effect of trace metals on male infertility

Metals are present in water, air, food, dietary supplements, alcoholic drinks and tobacco. Exposure to trace metals affects reproductive function and also affects the prostate function and serum testosterone concentration (Pizent *et al.*, 2012). Men are normally exposed to trace metals and other causative agents. All these together acts and cause the severe health defects. In human heavy toxic metals can disturb the necessary metal metabolism and decrease the metabolic functions (Matovic *et al.*, 2011). As a result of these improper cell growth, development, differentiation and affects the normal physiological action in organisms. Metals have a strong influence in genetic polymorphisms and many studies reported that heavy metals can change the triplet code for protein, as the result enzymes are produced with modified functions (Apostoli *et al.*, 2007).

Some of the trace elements like zinc, magnesium, calcium, sodium, potassium etc. have been essential for testicular development and spermatogenesis, are play an important in the physiology of spermatozoa (Tvrda *et al.*, 2015). But some of the heavy metals such as lead, mercury, chromium, copper, manganese, arsenic, iron directly linked with male fertility by decreasing semen quality, sub-fertility, and change in birth sex ratio, sexually transmitted infections, genito-urinary tract infections/inflammations, deficiencies of dietary antioxidant nutrients and an increase in the prevalence of developmental abnormalities of the male reproductive tract (Swan *et al.*, 2000). Many authors reported the concentration of heavy metals in seminal plasma to have a negative correlation with semen and sperm parameters (Hasan *et al.*, 2007 and Jeng *et al.*, 2015). Increasing the exposure to environmental chemicals that act endocrine gland disrupters were associated with semen quality (Pant *et al.*, 2013 & Wong and Cheng, 2011).

1.4.1 Role of calcium on male infertility

Calcium (Ca) is one of the most extensively studied elements of mammalian semen are calcium (Jensen *et al.*, 2016). Many research studies were conducted to examine the role of calcium in male infertility; the results of such studies produce conflicting data (Logoglu *et al.*, 1997). The seminal plasma concentration of calcium was observed the same in both fertile and infertile men (Umeyama *et al.*, 1986). There is no significance between the total calcium and seminal parameters, but poor motility was observed in men with low seminal plasma calcium concentration than men with normal motility (Prien *et al.*, 1990). Similarly, the seminal plasma calcium concentration of men with hypomotility was observed when compared to normal males (Wong *et al.*, 2001). Another study also suggested that the men with or without varicocele have lower calcium level than the fertile group (Hamada *et al.*, 2013). Other studies concluded those fertile groups have a high concentration of seminal plasma calcium than infertile group (Logoglu *et al.*, 1997). The exposure of the sperm *in vitro* medium containing low-level calcium shows a decrease in activity. It was known from the above study that low level of seminal plasma calcium leads to infertility (Nishida *et al.*, 1996). New studies have also illustrated that there is a close relationship between seminal calcium concentration and vitamin D (Jensen *et al.*, 2011). Calcium can regulate the sperm production, fertilization process, germ cell growth, differentiation, proliferation. Recent investigations have shown that calcium accumulation is seen in the certoli, myoid and leydig cells (Golpour *et al.*, 2017). Low concentration of seminal plasma calcium was observed in four infertile groups than in normozoospermic men (Bassey *et al.*, 2013).

1.4.2 Role of magnesium on male infertility

Magnesium (Mg) is an important cation found in all enzymatic function in the body. This cation has the capacity to modify the substrate of the enzyme and also act as a cofactor in more than 300 metabolic functions. Magnesium has a vital role in seminal parameters particularly in sperm motility; it is also used as a biomarker to identify the seminal vesicles secretions (Abou-Shakra *et al.*, 1989). A research study conducted to determine the role of blood and semen magnesium concentration of fertile and sub fertile males. Data obtained show that the blood concentrations of magnesium of fertile and sub fertile males do not have a significant difference but, there is a strong correlation in seminal plasma concentration between two groups (Wong *et al.*, 2001). Seminal plasma with a high concentration of magnesium may directly affect the fertilizing capacity, sperm production, maturation and motility (Skandhan, 1992). A data of the research study shows that the low concentration of magnesium in seminal plasma leads to premature ejaculation in both normal and infertile males (Omu *et al.*, 2001). An experimental study was conducted in 500 fertile and infertile males to investigate the correlation between the seminal plasma magnesium concentration and seminal parameters. Study results concluded that there is a strong negative correlation between the seminal plasma concentrations of magnesium and seminal parameters like sperm count, motility and morphology (Heidari, 2016). The relationship between seminal plasma magnesium levels with oxidative stress in Iraqi infertile men was studied and collected data conclude that the low-level magnesium was observed in oligozoospermic, azoospermic group compared to the normozoospermic group. Also, the high concentration of lipid peroxidation was recorded in all abnormal groups than the normal control group (Abdul-Rasheed, 2010).

1.4.3 Role of zinc on male infertility

Zinc (Zn) has various important physiological functions and during reproduction, it is needed for conception, implantation and positive pregnancy outcome. The human seminal fluid contains a high concentration of zinc and it has the wide role in sperm function. Globally many research studies reported the association of seminal plasma zinc and male infertility but show contradictory results. Few studies reported that seminal plasma zinc was observed less concentration in male with infertility problem than normal male (Turk *et al.*, 2014; Colagar *et al.*, 2009; Camejo *et al.*, 2011 and Hadwan *et al.*, 2012). During the early development of sperm, the zinc is accumulated in seminal plasma and sperm protein has zinc as a cofactor for its normal function (Elgazar *et al.*, 2005). Antibacterial activity and anti-lipid peroxidation property of zinc help to maintain sperm membrane and protect against degenerative changes in the testis (Eggert-Kruse *et al.*, 2002). Evidence reported that there is a change in fertilization due to the poor quality of semen when the participants with low concentrations of zinc (Colagar *et al.*, 2009). Increasing the sperm concentration during ejaculation, high motility, and increase antioxidant activity was observed when the seminal plasma has the optimal concentration of zinc (Oliva *et al.*, 2009). Role of zinc in semen parameters have been regulated due to the presence of high fatty layer in testis tissues lead to interfering with endocrine function (Merrells *et al.*, 2009). Zinc sulfate is used to reduce anti-sperm antibody (ASA) in the infertile male. The study results show that zinc sulfate treatment shows a significant enhancement of seminal parameters like concentration, count, motility and normal morphology (Jawad, 2013). A study was conducted to compare the seminal zinc concentration of fertile and infertile male with smoking/ nonsmoking habit. The result shows that zinc level was observed high in nonsmoker when compared to the smoker (Colagar *et al.*, 2009). A longitudinal study was conducted of infertile men treated with the zinc sulfate 200 mg capsule. Study data show that there is no significant increase in the serum zinc level before and after treatment, but there is gradually increase in seminal zinc concentration after treatment (Mossa *et al.*, 2011).

1.4.4 Role of sodium and potassium on male infertility

The metabolism, survival and function of sperm mainly happen in seminal plasma. Cations such as sodium (Na) and potassium (K) in the seminal plasma mainly to maintain osmotic balance and these also act as cofactors of many important enzymes. Thus to diagnose male infertility and other reproductive disorder the biochemical evaluation of seminal plasma is very important (Barrier-Battut *et al.*, 2002). Seminal plasma with a high concentration of sodium and potassium has been explained to be correlated with male infertility with poor semen quality. The seminal plasma concentration of Na and K are lower than intracellular concentration and thus sodium and potassium is linked to semen parameters. Higher concentrations of K are negatively impacting in ram sperm motility and show improvement in motility while treated with sodium chloride (Abdel-Rahman *et al.*, 2000). Mannowetz *et al.,* (2013), have shown that the potassium channel in human sperm is opened by increased levels of calcium ions inside the sperm cells.

1.4.5 Role of copper on male infertility

Copper (Cu) is an important trace element for the physiological functions of living organisms. Copper is also acting as a cofactor in many enzymatic reactions in the cell. Deficiency of copper in the human body can reduce the action of many enzymes and thereby interruption in many processes inside the cell. On the other side if the concentration is very high it can release of free radicals leads to damage of proteins and DNA. Foods like meat, nuts, legumes, seeds are the few major sources of copper (Morris *et al.*, 2006). Municipal garbage, agricultural chemicals, electrical items are the industrial sources of copper (Bertram *et al.*, 2002). Saleh *et al.*, (2008) explained that the copper concentration in azoospermic semen was observed low when compared to healthy males. Studies conducted on azoospermic patient's show that decrease in seminal copper concentrations leads to a decrease in superoxide dismutase (SOD) activity and also have a higher risk of oxidative stress. Akinloye *et al.*, (2011) reported that copper has shown positive effects on the volume of semen in both normal and abnormal patients. The concentration of blood and seminal copper shows positive correlation on sperm motility and count (Machal *et al.*, 2002). The animal with the copper deficiency ejaculate low volume of semen, less concentration of sperm with poor motility and show abnormal morphology. Due to inactive Sertoli cells, the seminiferous tubules were less developed. These abnormalities became normal after successful treatment with copper supplement (Van Niekerk *et al.*, 1989). Metabolic abnormalities, environmental pollution, and lifestyle changes are main factors lead to high accumulation of copper in human may directly or indirectly show the impact on male infertility (Letelier *et al.*, 2010). Few research studies show that a higher level of seminal copper shows a negative correlation with seminal parameters such as motility, viability and morphology (Eidi *et al.*, 2010 and Schmid *et al.*, 2013).

1.4.6 Role of chromium on male infertility

The reproductive system of men is highly sensitive to the environment and its factors show the effect to decrease the semen quality in a human being (Hernandez-Ochoa *et al.*, 2005 and Sharpe, 2010). Chromium (Cr) is present in the wide range of forms. Steel industries use chromium (0), whereas chromium (VI and III) are used in chrome plating, pigments, dyes, leather tanning, and also for wood preserving. Chromium occurs in the environment by naturally and also present as an essential nutrient in some food like broccoli (Pizent *et al.*, 2012). Chromium is an important metal plays an important role in glucose and fat metabolism. An excessive amount of chromium affect the reduction in oxidation, hydrolysis activity leads to denature of functional proteins and modified the general enzymatic reactions (Yu-gang *et al.*, 2006). Since it acts as cofactors for a wide range of vital enzymes, its concentration has associated with poor semen quality in rodents and also in humans (Meeker *et al.*, 2008). Lab animals and humans exposure to chromium (VI) has been reported to cause reproductive defects (Subramanian *et al.*, 2006). Male working in electroplating has poor semen quality with low sperm count and motility. Hormones like FSH of these participants were found in higher concentration (Multinger *et al.*, 1996). Chromium exposure can decrease the sperm count and increase the abnormal sperm in mice (Acharya *et al.*, 2006) rats (Li *et al.*, 2001) and rabbits (Yousef *et al.*, 2006). Animal study shows that male rat received potassium dichromate injection for 15 days decrease the testis weight and increase in seminal vesicles. The hormones like FSH got increased and LH got decreased in potassium dichromate treated rat (Marouani *et al.*, 2012).

1.4.7 Role of selenium on male infertility

Selenium (Se) is an important micronutrient in the diet for maintains a good reproductive health. There are only limited studies on the role of selenium in male reproduction. Hurst *et al.*, (1999) reported that infertile males have lower selenium level in the seminal plasma than the fertile male. From this study, it was concluded that selenium has a reasonable relationship with male infertility. Boitani and Puglisi, (2007) states that selenium is essential for normal sperm production in mammals and its function is mediated by two selenoproteins, namely phospholipid hydroperoxide glutathione peroxidase (PHGPx/GPx4) and Selenoprotein P. These selenoproteins are expressed in germ cells of the testis and have a wide range of function in the reproductive system. Foresta *et al.*, (2002) studied the relationship between male infertility and sperm PHGPx in 75 study subjects.

In a study conducted in Zagreb by Krsnjavi *et al.,* (1992), the effective role of selenium in male infertility from 18 males with poor semen quality and count. The author also studied the prevalence of male infertility with respect to age, smoking, alcohol and coffee. The study shows that selenium was significantly higher in control groups than in oligozoospermia and azoospermia group. Vezina *et al.*, (1996) conducted a study in Canada to examine the beneficial effect of selenium in infertile males. The entire study, patients received 400 mg of Vitamin E and 100 μg of selenium daily for one month. The dosage of vitamin E and selenium was gradually increased for 5 months. End of the study, there is a significant improvement in sperm motility, count and morphology. A research study conducted in 69 infertile Scottish male was treated with Selenium in a combination of vitamins like A, C and E for 90 days. All the participants showed significant improvement in sperm motility at the end of the clinical trial (Scott *et al.,* 1998). Various research studies conducted in worldwide to examine the role of selenium in the male infertility and also show the positive correlation of Se and semen parameters (Iwanier and Zachara, 1995 and Titan, 1992). Conception rates in cattle and secondary follicle formation in goats improved by selenium supplements (Kommisrud *et al.*, 2005 and Wu *et al.*, 2011). Testosterone production and sperm synthesis may change based on the concentration of selenium (Ahsan *et al.*, 2014).

1.4.8 Role of lead on male infertility

Many industrial chemicals are known to have a negative impact on human reproduction; various environmental and occupational exposures to toxic substance such as lead (Pb) are important reasons for male infertility (Sinclair, 2000). This chemical shows effect based on the concentration and duration of exposure. In simple if the lead concentration is high in blood for many years leads to severe damage to various tissues in the organisms. Epidemiological study on occupational exposure on male range more than 40 μg/dL has shown to increase the risk of male infertility or poor quality (Gennart *et al.*, 1992). A pilot study conducted in 4000 male workers with the high concentration of lead has shown a reduction in the number of children when compared to control group (Lin *et al.*, 1996). Animal studies have that lead is the one of the active element affect the male reproductive function (Nathan *et al.*, 1992). Studies conducted in many countries states that there is no association between low fertility rate and occupational exposure of lead (Joffe, 2003). A study conducted on lead battery workers was not able to confirm the effect of lead on male infertility in French (Coste *et al.*, 1991) and Danish population (Bonde and Kolstad, 1997).

Occupational lead exposure in men show wide range of seminal parameters affects like reduction in sperm count and density (Naha *et al.*, 2005), decrease in ejaculation volume and also correlation with asthenozoospermia, hypospermia and teratozoospermia (Lancranjan *et al.*, 1975) have been reported in male workers when the concentration at >40 μg/dL. High level of immature and abnormal sperm such as wide, round, short sperm was observed in workers who occupationally exposed to lead at high (40 μg/dL) (Telisman *et al.*, 2007). Animal studies show that when the male mice injected with lead acetate leads to reduction in the number of sperms within the epididymis and also regulated the sperm production in rats (Batra *et al.*, 2001). Lead can induce the sperm functional disorders like immature acrosome, unable to penetrate oocyte and also decrease the artificial insemination rates in human (Benoff *et al.*, 2003). The study reported that the semen lead concentration was negatively related to serum testosterone level among the occupationally exposed men (Alexander *et al.*, 1998). Additional evidence shows that the concentration of lipid peroxidation was observed high in the reproductive organs of rats were chronically exposed to lead (Marchlewicz *et al.*, 2007).

To evaluate the association of blood and seminal plasma lead with male infertility a case-control study was conducted in 52 males. Study results show that there is a positive significant correlation between semen and blood lead levels but there is no significant correlation with semen parameters and serum hormone concentration and lead concentration in this study population (Debnath and Fatima, 2010). Few studies reported that paternal lead exposure can affect the semen quality and delayed conception (Apostoli *et al.*, 2000 and Joffe *et al.*, 1999). A study conducted in Poland revealed that the percentage of couples with delayed conception were similar among the occupational exposed of lead and unexposed participants (Sitarek *et al.*, 1998). In the Danish study, exposure to lead on male infertility with respective age (cut off point at 30 years of age) was observed. Study result shows that reduced fertility was observed among the older age men than among the younger age men of battery workers (Bonde and Kolstad, 1997). When the lead concentration was observed at >40 μg/dL there is a decrease in semen quality parameters and also changes in the endocrine profile of the occupationally exposed participants (Viskum *et al.*, 1999).

1.5 Role of hormones on male infertility

Hormones are proteins, which play a vital role in initiating and maintaining the male reproductive system. Many studies have associated the level of hormones in blood serum with the quality of semen (Sina *et al.*, 1975; Subhan *et al.*, 1995; Jensen *et al.*, 1997 and Mahmoud *et al.*, 1998). Abnormal production of thyroid during testis development at a younger age has been shown an effect on testis maturation at reproductive age (Jannini *et al.*, 1995). FSH and LH have a synergic effect on the growth and protection of testicular function in males (Matsumoto *et al.*, 1983 & 1984). Studies reported that fertilization and pregnancy rate was improved in infertile male after administration of follicle stimulating hormone (FSH) (Acosta *et al.*, 1992). FSH is one of the main hormones in the male reproductive system and helps in sertoli and granulosa cells function, production of male gametes. Initiation of sperm production at puberty stage and maintain the healthy sperm production in the male based on the concentration of FSH (Tapanainen *et al.*, 1997). Higher levels of prolactin directly affect sexual system through a central nervous system and inhibit the production of androgen. The productions of testosterone by leydig cells are initiated through LH, which plays an important role in sperm production. Abnormal production of LH directly affects the sperm production lead to male infertility (Ramanujam *et al.*, 2000). A wide range of proteins such as estrogen, activin, follistatin and cytokines secreted locally have paracrine/autocrine regulation on sperm production. Similarly, other hormones leptin (Clement *et al.*, 1998), IGF-1 (Gnessi *et al.*, 1997), growth hormone (GH) (Hull and Harvey, 2000a), insulin-like growth factor-1 and thyroid hormone (Beamer *et al.*, 1981) are also been involved in sperm production. A hormonal concentration between the central nervous system and the testis control the sperm production. Imbalance in hormonal concentration has a negative impact on male infertility (Jarow, 2003).

1.6 Effect of environmental factors on male infertility

Male infertility caused by a variety of other factors which includes environmental (pollution, chemicals, etc.), lifestyle (smoking and chewing, alcohol, caffeine, some dietary components and some modern electronic gadgets etc.) and occupational (exposure of heavy metals, stress, high temperature etc.) factors. All the above said factors are affecting the male fertility by interfering with spermatogenesis, spermiogenesis, sperm motility, morphology, DNA, chromatin integrity and hormonal regulations or by reducing the fertilizing capacity of spermatozoa (Sharpe, 2000 and Ivell, 2007). The reproductive capacity of human is gradually reduced by various environmental agents. When the workers are exposed to various chemical and physical agents that are generated by industrial activities are the main causes of infertility (Slutsky *et al.*, 1999). Many studies in animals show that chemical classes of pesticide, insecticide and various solvents used in a wide range of industries are the potential reproductive toxicants (Sundaram and Witorsch, 1995). These substances have a strong influence on the production of sperm and many cross-sectional studies also stated that low infertility rate was observed in occupationally exposed population (Ratcliffe *et al.*, 1989). These hazardous chemicals directly damaged the testis of workers and results in low sperm count, abnormal sperm morphology (Bonde, 1996).

1.7 Effect of smoking on male infertility

Many studies report shows the negative impact of smoking on semen quality such as viability, sperm concentration, motility and morphology (Zhang *et al.*, 2000 and Kunzle *et al.*, 2003). A research study conducted by Sergerie *et al.*, (2000) found that sperm DNA is highly damaged in heavy smokers. Studies on the effect of smoking and male infertility found that smoking has a low influence on semen parameters (Marinelli *et al.*, 2004). Ramlau-Hansen *et al.*, (2006) documented an inverse dose-response relationship between smoking, semen volume, total sperm count and percentage of motile sperm. Another study showed that men with varicocele who smoked more than 10 cigarettes per day had impaired sperm motility and morphology (Collodel *et al.*, 2009). Many carcinogenic compounds found in a cigarette are directly entered in blood and found in seminal plasma. These compounds have directly induced the degradation of sperm and its quality. This leads to the low chance of pregnancy. They may also have a negative impact on the offspring and may develop childhood cancers (Sepaniak *et al.*, 2004). Smoking has directly influenced the hormonal level. The oestrone concentration level is found to be very high in smokers. Acrosin activity was decreased if the person smokes continually for 10 years and leads to infertile. Low acrosin activity sperm is not able to penetrate the oocyte and also have head morphology defects (Gerhardt *et al.*, 1989).

1.8 Effect of alcoholism on male infertility

Many research studies show that excessive alcohol consumption directly decreases the sperm count, changes in sperm morphology and it is the toxin to a testicular and leydig cell (Guo *et al.*, 2006). Men with alcohol habit are found a significant decrease in semen density, semen volume and sperm motility (Martini *et al.*, 2004). Seminal fluid of alcoholic user found to contain a high number of leukocytes than in nonalcoholic person (Close *et al.*, 1990). The hormonal concentration of alcoholic was significantly increased results in decreased motility, count and morphology (Muthusami and Chinnaswamy, 2005). Person consumes a high volume of alcohol result in abnormal testosterone production and the shrinkage of the testis (Adler, 1992). A clinical study shows that the excessive alcohol consumption not only decreases the testosterone production but it also alters the testosterone metabolism (Southren *et al.*, 1973). Researchers have proposed several mechanisms that may contribute to the alcohol-induced testosterone suppression (Anderson *et al.*, 1983). Libido and sexual potency of an advanced alcoholic were decreased and it's also noted that impotence was seen high in among the patients with liver damage (Lloyd and Williams, 1948). A recent systematic review and Meta analysis study shows that Intake of ethanol has a high impact on semen quality and authors suggest that persons planning to have a child must avoid excess consumption of ethanol (Ricci *et al.*, 2017). Absorption of zinc in the body is drastically reduced by excessive consumption of alcohol lead to zinc deficiency. Research studies shows that persons with low sperm count are found to have a zinc deficiency (Colagar *et al.*, 2009).

1.9 Effect of obesity on male infertility

Male become overweight and obese at reproductive age has been drastically increased over the past 30 years which leads to male infertility. Research studies show that male obesity has a direct impact on the male reproductive system with poor semen quality and also changes in germ cell morphology. Male obesity affects the child metabolism and the reproductive system by transmitting the paternal health issues to the next generation through sperm (Palmer *et al.*, 2012). According to WHO (1987), male with low and high BMI (less than 19 kg/m^2 or more than 30 kg/m^2, respectively) have low semen volume and poor semen quality (Jensen *et al.*, 2004). Men with high BMI produce only a low concentration of testosterone and leads to reduced fertility compared to men with normal weight (Sallmen *et al.*, 2006). Male obesity is suspected to cause alterations in semen parameters, especially sperm concentration, total sperm count, total motile sperm count, total progressively motile sperm count, sperm morphology and DNA fragmentation (Kort *et al.*, 2006 and MacDonald *et al.*, 2010).

1.10 Effect of diet on male infertility

Nutrition plays an important role in the male reproductive system. Animal and human research studies show that the intake of a high-fat diet may directly affect male infertility with poor semen quality and changes in sperm morphology. Diet with high energy fat like Tran's fatty acids and saturated fats directly affects the lipid metabolism in testis and cause an adverse effect on sperm production. High caloric diet increased the blood cholesterol level and cause obesity leads to a decrease in motility, inability to fertilize the egg and affect the sperm production in rabbits (Mitchell *et al.*, 2011; Palmer *et al.*, 2012; Rato *et al.*, 2013 and Morgan *et al.*, 2014). Due to lifestyle changes, men at reproductive age are changed their healthy eating habits. 70% of the male like to take junk foods and fried items instead of fruits and vegetables (Lioret *et al.*, 2012). Healthy diet nutrients rich in omega-3 fatty acids, vitamin E and C, beta-carotene, low saturated food items are good to maintain healthy sperm. Fruits, vegetables, skimmed milk, cereals and seafood were having the positive correlation with semen quality. Food items like potatoes, full-fat milk, cheese, excess coffee, beverages, sweets, and alcohol have also had an influence on semen quality and sperm production (Salas-Huetos *et al.*, 2017). Oleic acid and docosahexaenoic acid (DHA) concentration of seminal plasma were observed very low in normal patients (Conquer *et al.*, 1999). Results from the case-control study shows that the omega-3 fatty acid concentration in blood and seminal plasma were observed very high in healthy male than infertility male (Safarinejad *et al.*, 2010). Some of the research studies show that consumption of beef can alter the sperm morphology and semen quality (Swan *et al.*, 2007). Results show that the person having the habit of eating meat at very frequently was having poor semen quality (Braga *et al.*, 2012). Red meat intake has a negative correlation with semen parameters (Mendiola *et al.*, 2009); soy is a vegetable source for protein. Some studies shows that consuming soy have also influence in male infertility (Chavarro *et al.*, 2008), person with eating whole fruits and vegetable are lower risk of getting male infertility (Eslamian *et al.*, 2012). People are also using herbal plants from ancient times to treat male infertility (Mohajeri *et al.*, 2009). Intake of garlic powder for 70 days can increase the sperm count (Khaki *et al.*, 2011), carrot can enhance the production of male sex hormones (Nouri *et al.*, 2009), ginger have property to protect sperm DNA damage (Khaki *et al.*, 2009), oral administration of Cinnamomum increased the weight of the testis and improved semen quality (Shalaby and Mouneir, 2010). The antioxidant effect of fenugreek seed enriches the semen quality and sperm motility (Kaviarasan *et al.*, 2007). Libido, semen quality, the concentration of testosterone was improved by intake of pumpkin seed and its oil which contain essential fatty acids (Bjorbaek and Kahn, 2004). A number of herbal medicines have a positive correlation with semen parameters (count, viability and motility), decreasing the abnormal sperm, induce the sexual desire (erection, intromission and ejaculating capacity) (Mohammadi *et al.*, 2013).

1.11 Role of vitamin D on male infertility

Vitamin D is an important molecule with multifunctional and involved in autocrine, paracrine and endocrine systems. It is also mediated in genomic actions and target in many organs and systems in the human body. The role of the vitamin in male infertility which includes sperm production, sex hormone synthesis has been studied in animal and humans and explained about the beneficial effect on male infertility (de Angelis *et al.*, 2017). Several parts of reproductive system have vitamin D receptor shows the positive correlation with male infertility (Jensen *et al.*, 2011). Recent studies reported a relationship between vitamin D and poor semen quality in infertile men (Tak *et al.*, 2015). In addition, an association between vitamin D and serum androgen has been reported (Wehr *et al.*, 2010). In recent years, there has been a growing interest in studying the association of vitamin D deficiency and infertility (Li *et al.*, 2012). Vitamin D is absorbed by Vitamin D Receptors (VDR) which is present in the surface of the cells. Many research studies were reported that VDR was observed in tissues present in the reproductive organ. Research studies conducted to explain the positive correlation of vitamin D with seminal parameters. Vitamin D involved enzymes were seen in mature sperm, human testis and in ejaculatory tract which conclude that the vitamin D is necessary for sperm production and maturation (Firouzabadi *et al.*, 2014; Rudick *et al.*, 2012; Garbedian *et al.*, 2013 and Paffoni *et al.*, 2014). A cross-sectional study conducted in 300 participants, which shows that lower concentration of serum vitamin D significantly reduced the number and motility of sperm (Jensen *et al.*, 2018). A prospective study of sperm collected from fertile men to determine the VDR in human sperm by Immunoassay, results show that the receptor of Vitamin D proved to present in Head, Midpiece and tail of the sperm. This is the first study identified the presence of VDR in human sperm (Corbett *et al.*, 2006). A case-control study was conducted in idiopathic male infertility to analysis the vitamin D treatment and male infertility. The result shows that lower concentration of vitamin D in serum and semen was observed in the study population. There is a significant improvement in sperm count, motility and morphology after successful vitamin D treatment. Thus vitamin D supplement has confirmed to enhance the semen parameters (Alzoubi *et al.*, 2017).

1.12 DNA fragmentation and male infertility

Apart from the normal semen parameters used to diagnose male infertility, now it is important to analyze the sperm DNA (Deoxy ribonucleic acid) by using modern techniques to find the real reasons for male infertility. Sperm DNA integrity is very important to maintain the normal reproductive function. To achieve the pregnancy it's not only important of sperm motility and function but also the DNA integrity is important for normal embryo and fetal growth (Sharma *et al.*, 2004). Male show normal sperm parameters may still infertile due to the loss of DNA integrity. Oocyte fertilized with sperm contain abnormal DNA may not develop normally, therefore it is very important to analyze the DNA of sperm along with normal semen parameters to avoid future problems. Suitable sperm DNA assay explains not only the power of sperm to fertilize but also help doctors to select the choice of treatment to achieve pregnancy (Perreault *et al.*, 2003). A number of research studies reported that the sperm DNA damage have the negative effects on the semen parameters such as morphology, motility (Giwercman *et al.*, 2003 and McVicar *et al.*, 2004). Few studies conducted on different population used a wide range of DNA assays found that semen parameters have a strong relationship with DNA nature, whereas few found no such associations (Henkel *et al.*, 2003). Sperm Chromatin Structure Assay (SCSA) (Evenson *et al.*, 2002), the Terminal deoxynucleotidyl transferase dUTP nick end labelling (TUNEL) assay, the In Situ Nick Translation (ISNT) (Gorczyca *et al.*, 1993), the DNA Breakage Detection-Fluorescence in Situ Hybridization (DBD-FISH) test (Fernandez *et al.*, 2002), the Comet Assay (Fernandez *et al.*, 2003), the single-cell pulsed-field gel electrophoresis technique (Kaneko *et al.*, 2012) and the Sperm Chromatin Dispersion Test (SCDt) (Lewis *et al.*, 2008 and Gosalvez *et al.*, 2008) are few commonly used assays to determine the sperm DNA damage. A study conducted on the Algerian population on male infertility shows that the semen parameters have negatively correlated with sperm DNA damage (Boushaba and Belaaloui, 2015). A recent study conducted to examine the relationship between the semen parameters and DNA damage in 203 participants who came for IVF treatment. The study results show that the IVF group participants with <25% sperm DFI (DNA Fragments Integrity) had a 33% birth rate while participants with >50% DFI had only 13% birth rate (Simon *et al.*, 2013). In Meta-analysis study the pregnancy success rate is significantly increased in participants with low sperm DFI compared to those with high sperm DFI (Osman *et al.*, 2015). Many research studies conducted in recent years reported that Oxidative stress (OS) is one of the risk factors that affect the sperm dysfunction (Tesarik *et al.*, 2006) and DNA damage (Loft *et al.*, 2003). Wide range of DNA damage such as DNA strand breaks and base oxidation, chromatin cross-linking, chromosome deletion and mediate apoptosis are caused by OS (Said *et al.*, 2004). OS is directly increasing the abnormal sperm (Gil-Guzman *et al.*, 2001), which have a negative correlation in fertilization capacity and IVF success rate *in vivo* (Zorn *et al.,* 2003). In ICSI, the embryo is not able to reach the blastula stage when it fertilizes by sperm with damaged DNA (Nasr-Esfahani *et al.,* 2005). Studies proved that high level of sperm DNA fragmentation (SDF) was observed in infertile men with varicocele, also confirmed that there is a decent improvement in SDF, semen parameters and increase the pregnancy rate at post varicocelectomy (Wang *et al.*, 2012). The success rate of ART is reduced due to the presence of SDF. A study conducted in Dakar to study the association of SDF and ART success rate result shows that the SDF index was higher in participants with fertility problem than in control groups (Diallo *et al.*, 2015).

2.0 OBJECTIVE OF THE PRESENT STUDY

1. The present study has been designed to examine the level of toxicity of trace metals on human semen quality. Trace metals are commonly observed in the natural environment with highly contaminated and these have been suggested as being very toxic to the human physiological process. This would facilitate examination of the role of these toxic trace metals in the alternation of various semen parameters such as count, motility, morphology, hormones concentration and DNA damage.

2. The main objective of the current study was also to examine the relationship between the trace metals and prevalence of male infertility in and around Chennai, Tamilnadu, India. The study also endeavors to determine the occupational exposure of trace metals in study participants and trace metal concentration on seminal plasma.

3. An attempt has also been made to assess the concentration of serum hormones, vitamin D and its correlation with semen quality in study participants. Hormone profiles which includes thyroid stimulating hormone (TSH), follicle-stimulating hormone (FSH), luteinizing hormone (LH), prolactin (PRL) and testosterone (TST) levels in the infertile men was also focused.

4. Apart from the regular semen analysis in this present study the percentage of sperm DNA damage is analysed in all study participants and compared with the semen quality.

Therefore the objective of the current work was to establish semen variables as effective tool and trace metals used as seminal biomarkers which may cause reproductive dysfunction in humans.

3.0 EXPERIMENTAL METHODS

3.1 Study area

This research study was conducted at the Department of Andrology, Kanmani Fertility Centre Pvt. Ltd., Chennai, Tamilnadu, India. The methodology and protocol of the present study was approved by Institutional Ethical Committee, The New College, Chennai and the informal consent was obtained by the individual participant.

3.2 Study sample size

A total of 60 infertile men from South India, Tamilnadu, were participated in this study. Sample size was calculated using sample size determination in health studies formula and a prevalence of 10% (Lwanga and Lemeshow, 1991).

3.3 Inclusion criteria

Healthy male subjects aged between 20 and 50 years, who had history of infertility for more than one year and who sought treatment for infertility from the Kanmani Fertility Centre Pvt. Ltd., Chennai, Tamilnadu, India were included.

3.4 Data collection

Data collection was made through the questionnaire which includes age, marital status, infertility duration, family history, occupation, lifestyle, environmental factors, medical histories, health problems and parity. Mainly a history of trace metals exposure or resided in areas known to have a trace metal contaminations, alcoholic consumption, and smoking and tobacco usage were considered.

3.5 Semen analysis

3.5.1 Semen collection

The participants were advised to collect the semen sample in a separate room near to the analytical lab by masturbation and the ejaculate was collected into sterile wide mouth container. Lab technician use to get all information from the patients regarding the collection methods and loss of any fraction of the sample. The sample container was marked with participant name, study id, semen collection, date, time and ethics number. Semen analysis was carried out as per WHO guidelines (WHO, 2010).

3.5.2 Liquefaction time

The collected semen samples was kept undisturbed in room temperature for 15–30 minutes for liquefaction before starting the microscopic examination and time taken for liquefaction was recorded.

3.5.3 Viscosity

The collected sample was examined for the viscosity by inserting the sterile glass rod in the sample tube and measuring the length of the thread that forms on withdrawal of the rod. Based on the consistency of the liquefied sample the viscosity was measured.

3.5.4 Volume and pH

The collected semen sample was carefully transferred into a graduated sterile glass tube to measure volume of the sample. The pH of the collected sample was measured by using pH paper.

3.5.5 Microscopic examinations

The semen quality which comprises the sperm concentration, motility, morphology and appearance of other cellular elements apart from spermatozoa was analyzed using microscope. About 10 μL of collected semen sample was applied to a clean glass slide and covered with a cover slip without any stain. The prepared slide was kept undisturbed for one minute for stabilization. A simple light microscope was used in this study for analyzing the semen parameters at a magnification of 20X and 40X. The appearance of other cells like epithelial cells, leucocytes, red blood corpuscles and immature germ cells were observed using the prepared wet slide. The number of sperm cells were calculated using the same wet slide, concentration of sperm was calculated in millions/mL and motility was calculated in percentage.

3.5.6 Sperm motility and viability

The motility of the sperm within the collected semen was examined immediately after liquefaction of the semen sample. The sample was mixed well without any air bubbles to avoid sedimentation of spermatozoa. The homogenous sample was used to prepare wet slides with 20 mm cover slip, which allow sperm swim freely. The slides were examined under microscopically at 20X and 40X magnifications to assess the different grades like progressive motility (PR), non-progressive motility (NP) and immotility (IM). The motility of sperm was calculated in percentage (%). The sperm viability was also examined by Eosin-Nigrosin method.

3.5.7 Sperm concentration

The hemocytometer was used to examine the concentration of sperm in the semen sample. 50 μL of well mixed liquefied semen sample was mixed with 950 μL of the semen diluting fluid (Diluting fluid: 10 mL of 35% formalin mixed with 50 g of sodium bicarbonate. After through dissolution of sodium bicarbonate, 5 mL of aqueous gentian violet was added and the resulting solution was made to a final volume of 100 mL). A small drop of diluted sample was applied in hemocytometer and covered with a cover slip. The concentration of sperm was counted after 5 minutes in the central square of the chamber using light microscope at 20X and 40X. The concentration of sperm was calculated as million/mL of the semen sample.

3.5.8 Sperm morphology

The morphology of sperm which includes, defects of sperm head (amorphous, tapering, swollen, vacuolated, large, small and double head), mid-piece (absent of mid-piece, thin and bend mid-piece) and tail (hairpin, broken, irregular, coiled and multiple) were observed in wet preparation slide stained with Papanicolaou method.

Staining procedure

1. Semen smear was prepared in clean glass slide and dried in air for 10 minutes at room temperature.
2. Air dried smear was kept in fixative for 30 minutes and allowed to dry.
3. The smear was dipped for 10 times in ethanol prepared its various concentration.
4. The smear was stained in Harris hematoxylin for 3 minutes and 2 dipped in distilled water.
5. The smear was dipped few times in acid-ethanol and finally rinsed with running water for 3–5 minutes.

6. The smear was further kept in a jar containing Scott's solution for about 4 minutes and washed in distilled water.

7. The smear was then dehydrated by dipping 10 times in 50%, 70%, 80%, 95% and 99.5% ethanol solutions.

8. The smear was first stained with orange G6 for 2 minutes followed by 95% ethanol wash.

9. The smear was stained with EA-50 for 5 minutes followed by 95% ethanol wash.

10. Finally the smear was kept in xylene for one minute and mounted in DPX.

11. The prepared smear slide was observed under light microscope at 100X for sperm morphology examination.

12. Minimum 100 sperms were counted in each smear to calculate the average percentage of sperms with abnormal morphology and different stages of immature sperm cells in the collected semen sample.

3.6 Estimation of trace metals

The following protocols were used to determine the metal ions in the seminal plasma. The reagents for calcium, magnesium, zinc, sodium, potassium and copper were purchased from Coral Clinical Systems, Tulip Group, Chennai, Tamilnadu, India.

3.6.1 Determination of seminal plasma calcium (Katayama *et al.*, 2013)

Principle:

Calcium gives a purple colour complex with o-cresolphthalein in an alkaline pH. The intensity of the colour is directly proportional to the amount of calcium present in the given semen sample.

Procedure

1. The seminal plasma calcium was estimated by spectrophotometric method.

2. Standard: 0.5 mL of working reagent mixed with 0.5 mL of coloured reagent and 0.02 mL of standard magnesium solution, incubated at 25 °C for 5 minutes.

3. Test: 0.5 mL of working reagent mixed with 0.5 mL of coloured reagent and 0.02 mL of seminal plasma, incubated at 25 °C for 5 minutes.

4. Blank: 0.5 mL of working reagent mixed with 0.5 mL of coloured reagent and 0.02 mL of distilled water, incubated at 25 °C for 5 minutes.

5. The absorbance of standard and test samples were recorded by using spectrophotometer at 570 nm yellow filter against the blank.

6. The calcium concentration in seminal plasma was calculated from the calibration curve.

Calculation

$$\text{Calcium (mg/dL)} = \frac{\text{Absorbance of sample}}{\text{Absorbance of standard}} \times \text{Concentration of standard (10 mg/dL)}$$

3.6.2 Determination of seminal plasma magnesium (Katayama *et al.*, 2013)

Principle:

Magnesium mixed with calmagite in an alkaline pH forms a red coloured solution. Obstruction of proteins and calcium is avoided by adding of specific chelating agents and detergents. The intensity of colour of the solution is directly proportional to amount of magnesium in the given semen sample.

Procedure

1. The seminal plasma magnesium was estimated by spectrophotometric method.

2. Standard: 0.5 mL of working reagent mixed with 0.5 mL of coloured reagent and 0.01 mL of standard magnesium solution, incubated at 25 °C for 5 minutes.

3. Test: 0.5 mL of working reagent mixed with 0.5 mL of coloured reagent and 0.01 mL of seminal plasma, incubated at 25 °C for 5 minutes.

4. Blank: 0.5 mL of working reagent mixed with 0.5 mL of coloured reagent and 0.01 mL of distilled water, incubated at 25 °C for 5 minutes.

5. The absorbance of standard and test samples were recorded by using spectrophotometer at 510 nm green filter against the blank.

6. The concentration of magnesium was determined by using calibration curve.

Calculation

$$\text{Magnesium (mEq/L)} = \frac{\text{Absorbance of sample}}{\text{Absorbance of standard}} \times \text{Concentration of standard (2 mEq/L)}$$

3.6.3 Determination of seminal plasma zinc (Makino *et al.*, 1991)

Principle:

Zinc reacts with Nitro-PAPS in an alkaline pH gives a purple coloured complex. The intensity of colour is directly proportional to the amount of zinc present in the given semen sample.

Procedure

1. The seminal plasma zinc was estimated by nitro-PAPS method.
2. Standard: 1 mL of zinc working reagent and 0.05 mL of standard solution was mixed and incubated at (25 °C) for 5 min.
3. Test: 1 mL of zinc working reagent and 0.05 mL of seminal plasma were mixed well and incubated at (25 °C) for 5 min.
4. Blank: 1 mL of zinc working reagent and 0.05 mL of distilled water were mixed well and incubated at (25 °C) for 5 min.
5. The absorbance of standard and test samples were recorded against the blank within 20 min by using spectrophotometer at 570 nm (yellow filter).
6. The concentration of zinc in sample was calculated from the calibration curve.

Calculation

$$\text{Zinc (}\mu\text{g/dL)} = \frac{\text{Absorbance of sample}}{\text{Absorbance of standard}} \times \text{Concentration of standard (200 }\mu\text{g/dL)}$$

3.6.4 Determination of seminal plasma sodium and potassium (Katayama *et al.*, 2013)

Sodium and potassium ions were determined on the basis of ion selective electrode method (ISE). Seminal plasma samples were collected and analyzed using direct ISE analyzer (Elite-3i, Tulip Diagnostics, India). Standard operating procedure was adopted during sample collection to avoid pre-analytical errors. The auto-analyzer was routinely calibrated every 24 hours by linear calibration. The concentration of sodium and potassium are expressed in mEq/L.

3.6.5 Determination of seminal plasma copper (Katayama *et al.*, 2013)

Principle:

Copper reacts with Di-Br-PAESA in acidic pH resulting a blue coloured complex. The concentration of copper in the give semen sample was calculated by the intensity of the coloured complex.

Procedure

1. The seminal plasma copper was estimated by spectrophotometer Di-Br-PAESA method.
2. Standard: 0.5 mL of working buffer reagent was mixed with 0.5 mL of colour reagent and 0.05 mL of standard copper solution, incubated at 25 °C for 10 min.
3. Test: 0.5 mL of working buffer reagent was mixed with 0.5 mL of colour reagent and 0.05 mL of seminal plasma, incubated at 25 °C for 10 min.
4. Blank: 0.5 mL of working buffer reagent was mixed with 0.5 mL of colour reagent and 0.05 mL of distilled water, incubated at 25 °C for 10 min.
5. The absorbance of standard and test samples were recorded against the blank within 30 min by using spectrophotometer at 580 nm (yellow filter).
6. The concentration of copper metal ion was calculated using calibration curve.

Calculation

$$\text{Copper } (\mu\text{g/dL}) = \frac{\text{Absorbance of sample}}{\text{Absorbance of standard}} \times \text{Concentration of standard } (200\ \mu\text{g/dL})$$

3.6.6 Determination of chromium, selenium and lead (Katayama *et al.*, 2013)

Amount of chromium, selenium and lead in seminal plasma was estimated by electro thermal atomic absorption spectrophotometer. Approximately 100 μL of seminal plasma sample was treated with 500 μL of super-grade 0.8M HNO_3 in a reaction tube. The mixture was dissolved in 1 mL of 1% HNO_3 which was applied to a graphite tube for the estimation of lead, chromium and selenium. The recovery of lead, chromium and selenium in spiked semen samples was 97%. The instrument was calibrated using 0 μg/L, 50 μg/L, 100 μg/L and 200 μg/L standards for lead chromium and selenium, respectively. A sample blank was prepared each time to avoid possible metal contamination from external sources. The instrument was allowed to analyse sample and display the concentration in μg/L.

3.7 Hormonal assay

Fasting venous blood samples were obtained from study subjects. Serum samples were separated by centrifugation at 3000 rpm for 15 min, and stored at –20 °C until the time of analysis. Serum levels of thyroid stimulating hormone (TSH), follicle stimulating hormone (FSH), luteinizing hormone (LH), prolactin (PRL), testosterone (TST) and vitamin D, were measured using Beckmen coulter access 2 (Electro-chemiluminescence immunoassay (ECLIA).

3.7.1 Estimation of thyroid stimulating hormone (TSH) (Sarkar, 2014)

Principle:

The serum hTSH binds with anti-hTSH, which is coated on the solid phase. The enzyme catalyst goat anti-hTSH-alkaline phosphatase conjugate the reaction and the non-reacted enzyme is removed by washing. A light is generated when the chemiluminescent substrate, Lumi-Phos 530 is added to the reaction vessels. The intensity of light is measured by Luminometer. The light production is directly proportional to the concentration of thyroid stimulating hormone in the sample.

Procedure

1. All the reagents were mixed well before processing in to the system.
2. The ready pack reagent is added in the primary reagent area.
3. The system automatically mixes the working reagents to maintain homogenous suspension and 200 μL of sample is loaded in the cuvette.
4. The serum sample container is arranged into to running rack with proper barcode and run the test.
5. 50 μL of lite reagent and 225 μL of solid phase were added, and the rack is incubated for 7.5 minutes at 37 °C
6. Washed the cuvettes with reagent water 300 μL each of acid reagent and base reagent to initiate the chemiluminescent reaction.
7. A direct relationship is obtained between the amount of TSH present in the patient sample and the amount of relative light units (RLUs) detected by the system.

Calculation

Serum TSH results were expressed in μIU/mL.

3.7.2 Estimation of follicle stimulating hormone (FSH) (Sarkar, 2014)

Principle:

The serum sample reacts with mouse anti-hFSH complexes and TRIS buffered saline with protein. The hFSH binds to the immobilized mouse anti-hFSH on the solid phase. The unbound materials are washed away. An enzyme alkaline phosphatase conjugated goat anti-hFSH is then added and binds to the previously bound hFSH on the particles and the unbound materials are washed away. The chemiluminescent substrate is added to the vessel, as the result of the reaction the light is generated which is measured with a Luminometer. The light intensity is directly proportional to the amount of hFSH in the sample.

Procedure

1. All the reagents are mixed well before processing in to the system.

2. The ready pack reagent is added in the primary reagent area.

3. The system automatically mixes the working reagents to maintain homogenous suspension and 200 µL of sample is loaded in the sample container.

4. The serum sample container is arranged into to running rack with proper barcode and run the test.

5. 100 µL of lite reagent (R1a) was added and incubates for 2.5 minutes at 37 °C separates, aspirates, and washes the cuvettes with wash buffer.

6. 400 µL of solid phase (R1b) was added and incubates for 2.5 minutes at 37 °C washes the cuvettes with wash buffer.

7. 300 µL each of acid reagent and base reagent (R1c) were added to initiate the chemiluminescent reaction. The results were read automatically after the end of reaction.

8. A direct relationship exists between the amount of FSH present in the patient sample and the amount of relative light units (RLUs) detected by the system.

Calculation

Serum FSH results were expressed in mIU/mL.

3.7.3 Estimation of luteinizing hormone (LH) (Sarkar, 2014)

Principle:

The serum sample reacts with mouse anti-hLH complexes and TRIS buffered saline with protein. The hLH binds to the immobilized mouse anti-hLH on the solid phase. The unbound materials are washed away. An enzyme alkaline phosphatase conjugated goat anti-hLH is then added and binds to the previously bound hLH on the particles and the unbound materials are washed away. The chemiluminescent substrate is added to the vessel, as the result of the reaction the light is generated which is measured with a luminometer. The light intensity is directly proportional to the amount of hLH in the sample.

Procedure

1. All the reagents are mixed well before processing in to the system.
2. The ready pack reagent is added in the primary reagent area.
3. The system automatically mixes the working reagents to maintain homogenous suspension and 200 µL of sample is loaded in the sample container.
4. The serum sample container is arranged into to running rack with proper barcode and run the test.
5. 100 µL of lite reagent (R1a) was added and incubates for 5.0 minutes at 37 °C separates, aspirates, and washes the cuvettes with wash buffer.
6. 400 µL of solid phase (R1b) was added and incubates for 2.5 minutes at 37°C washes the cuvettes with wash buffer.
7. 300 µL each of acid reagent and base reagent (R1c) were added to initiate the chemiluminescent reaction. Read the results automatically after the end of reaction.
8. A direct relationship exists between the amount of FSH present in the patient sample and the amount of relative light units (RLUs) detected by the system.

Calculation

Serum LH results were expressed in mIU/mL.

3.7.4 Estimation of prolactin (PRL) (Szosland, *et al.*, 2015)

Principle:

A serum sample mix with polyclonal goat anti-PRL alkaline phosphatase conjugate along with paramagnetic particles coated with mouse monoclonal anti-PRL antibody in the reaction vessel. The serum PRL binds with anti-PRL with the help of goat anti-PRL-alkaline phosphatase. A light is generated as the results of formation of antigen-antibody complex. The light produced is directly proportional to the concentration of prolactin in the given serum sample.

Procedure

1. All the reagents are mixed well before processing in to the system.
2. The ready pack reagent is added in the primary reagent area.
3. The system automatically mixes the working reagents to maintain homogenous suspension and 200 μL of sample is loaded in the sample container.
4. The serum sample container is arranged into to running rack with proper barcode and run the test.
5. 100 μL of lite reagent (R1a) was added and incubates for 5.0 minutes at 37 °C separates, aspirates, and washes the cuvettes with wash buffer.
6. 400 μL of solid phase (R1b) was added and incubated for 2.5 minutes at 37 °C washes the cuvettes with wash buffer.
7. 300 μL each of acid reagent and base reagent (R1c) were added to initiate the chemiluminescent reaction. Read the results automatically after the end of reaction.
8. A direct relationship exists between the amount of PRL present in the patient sample and the amount of relative light units (RLUs) detected by the system.

Calculation

Serum PRL results were expressed in ng/mL.

3.7.5 Estimation of testosterone (TST) (Niki *et al.,* 2014)

Principle:

The serum sample mix with sample treatment solution, mouse monoclonal anti-testosterone antibody, testosterone alkaline phosphatase conjugate, and paramagnetic particles coated with goat anti-mouse polyclonal antibody forms the antigen-antibody complex. The unbound materials are washed away after incubation. A light is generated as the result of antigen antibody complex which is read by Luminometer. The amount of testosterone is calculated by the intensity of the light.

Procedure

1. All the reagents are mixed well before processing in to the system.
2. The ready pack reagent is added in the primary reagent area.
3. The system automatically mixes the working reagents to maintain homogenous suspension and 100 µL of sample is loaded in the sample container.
4. The serum sample container is arranged into to running rack with proper barcode and run the test.
5. 50 µL of lite reagent (R1a) was added and incubates for 5.0 minutes at 37 °C separates, aspirates, and wash the cuvettes with wash buffer.
6. 300 µL of solid phase (R1b) was added and incubates for 5.0 minutes at 37 °C wash the cuvettes with wash buffer.
7. 300 µL each of acid reagent and base reagent (R1c) were added to initiate the chemiluminescent reaction. Read the results automatically after the end of reaction
8. A direct relationship exists between the amount of testosterone present in the patient sample and the amount of relative light units (RLUs) detected by the system.

Calculation

Serum testosterone results were expressed in ng/dL.

3.8 Estimation of vitamin D (Abbasihormozi *et al.*, 2017)

Principle:

In a reaction vessel the serum sample mix with a DBP releasing agent and paramagnetic particles coated with sheep monoclonal anti-vitamin D antibody. DBP release the vitamin D and binds with immobilized monoclonal anti-vitamin D in the presence of analogue-alkaline phosphatase. The reaction vessel is washes to remove unbound materials. An antigen-antibody complex is formed after the addition of chemiluminescent substrate Lumi-Phos 530. As a result the light is generated was measured using Luminometer. The light production is inversely proportional to the concentration of vitamin D present in the sample.

Procedure

1. All the reagents are mixed well before processing in to the system.

2. The ready pack reagent is added in the primary reagent area.

3. The system automatically mixes the working reagents to maintain homogenous suspension and 30 µL of sample is loaded in the sample container.

4. The serum sample container is arranged into to running rack with proper barcode and run the test.

5. 200 µL of ancillary pack reagent (R1a) was added and incubates for 4.5 minutes at 37 °C separates, aspirates, and wash the cuvettes with wash buffer.

6. 50 µL of solid phase (R1b) was added and incubates for 5.5 minutes at 37 °C wash the cuvettes with wash buffer.

7. 100 µL each of acid reagent and base reagent (R1c) were added 50 µL of ancillary well reagent to initiate the chemiluminescent reaction by incubation 2.75 minutes at 37 °C.

8. Read the results automatically after the end of reaction.

9. The amount of light production is inversely proportional to the amount of vitamin D present in the sample and the amount of relative light units (RLUs) detected by the system.

Calculation

Serum vitamin D results were expressed in ng/mL.

3.9 Examination/Assessment of sperm DNA fragmentation (Fernandez *et al.*, 2005).

The normality of sperm chromatin and DNA in study population was analysed using DNA fragmentation assay. Dyes like aniline blue, acridine orange, chromomycin used in this procedure to bind histone or nucleic acid and are histologically or flow cytometry used to assed the DNA fragmentation. Assessment of DNA strand breaks by terminal deoxynucleotidyl transferase (TdT)-mediated deoxyuridine triphosphate (dUTP)-nick-end labelling (or TUNEL for short (in situ end-labelling, ISEL)), comet assays or sperm chromatin dispersion (SCD). This procedure helps to get an additional information about fertilization rates with standard IVF and, possibly, spontaneous pregnancy rates. The sperm chromatin dispersion assay (SCD) can be predictive of fertilization failure *in vivo* and *in vitro*. The kits were commercially purchased from SAR Health Line Pvt. Ltd., Chennai, Tamilnadu, India.

Sample preparation

The collected semen sample was allowed to get liquefy at 37 °C and counted. The sample was diluted with PBS or sperm preparation media to make a final concentration about 15–20 million/mL.

Slide preparation

The agarose gel was melted at 90 °C for 5 minutes in sperm chroma warmer-1 and then the gel was transfer to sperm chroma warmer-2 to maintain at 37 °C for 5 minutes. 40 μL of sample was applied to agarose gel through micro pipette. The gel was mixed gently to avoid bubble formation. 150 μL of suspension was added on the coated slide and covered with provided coverslip. The slide was then transferred to 4–8 °C for 5 minutes for solidification and then the cover slip was removed carefully from the slide. 1 mL of acid denaturant was applied on the slide by keeping the slide in flat surface. The slide was incubated at 37 °C for 7 minutes and the excess solution was removed after incubation. 1 mL of lysis solution was applied on to the slide and incubated for 20 minutes. Excess lysis solution was removed after incubation. The slide was kept slanted position and washed with distilled water. The slide was dehydrated by using 1 mL of dehydrating solution1 followed by dehydrating solution-2 and dehydrating solution-3 and incubates for 5 minutes each. Finally the prepared slide was air dried and stored in dark at room temperature until further process.

Staining

300 μL of stain solution was mixed with 100 μL of dilution buffer in the dilution tube. The solution was mixed well and used within the hour of preparation.

Procedure

250 μL of freshly prepared working stain solution was applied carefully on to the slide and the stained was distributed uniformly. The slide was washed in water after 3 minutes of incubation and air dried. Finally the slide was observed under 20X and 40X of bright field microscope.

Calculation

Calculation of sperm DNA fragmentation (SDFI) value is done as followed.

$$\text{SDFI value (\%)} = \frac{\text{Number of Fragmented sperms}}{\text{Total number of sperms scored}} \times 100$$

3.10 Statistical Analysis

The experiments conducted in triplicates in this study were subjected to various statistical analyses using SPSS software that the standard error mean and P value significance were estimated and the results were inferred for logical interpretations.

4.0 RESULTS AND DISCUSSION

A total number of 100 participants who visited to Kanmani Fertility Center Pvt. Ltd., Chennai, Tamilnadu, India for fertility problem were asked the consent to participate, but only 60 participants were willing to enroll into the study. Based on semen parameters include sperm count, motility and morphology, the enrolled study participants were grouped into five categories (**Table 3 & Fig 1**), namely normozoospermia (15.0%), asthenozoospermia (26.6%), asthenoteratozoospermia (21.6%), oligoasthenozoospermia (16.6%), oligoasthenoteratozoospermia (20.0).

Group 1: Normozoospermia

Infertile participants have more than 15 million/mL of sperms in semen without any motility and morphological changes.

Group 2: Asthenozoospermia

Infertile participants have higher level of immotile sperm compared with normal.

Group 3: Asthenoteratozoospermia

Infertile participants have higher level of non-motile sperm and abnormal morphology compared with normal.

Group 4: Oligoasthenozoospermia

Infertile participants have lower level of sperm count (<15 million/mL) and reduced motility than normal level.

Group 5: Oligoasthenoteratozoospermia

Infertile participants with lower level of sperm count, sperm motility and abnormal morphology compared with normal.

4.1.3 Semen Volume

Data from **Table 4** show that the mean volume of semen was 4.1 mL, 3.2 mL, 3.0 mL, 3.7 mL and 2.8 mL for the groups 1–5, respectively. The lowest mean semen volume was noted in group 5 (2.8 mL) and the highest volume was found in group 1 (4.1 mL) (**Figure 3**). The semen volume ranged from 1.2 mL to 7.8 mL in group 1; 1.0 mL to 6.2 mL in group 2; 1.4 mL to 6.2 mL in group 3; 1.4 to 8.0 mL in group 4 and 1.4 mL to 4.8 mL in group 5 participants, respectively. Studies reported that various factors may influence the volume of semen. Marconi *et al.*, (2009) stated that male track infection is one of the main factors for lowering the semen levels. Study (Comhaire *et al.*, 1994) has shown that semen volume is one of the best indicators of *in vivo* fertilization capacity, which supports our results that apart from group 1 all other group participants were with low semen levels. Lifestyle factors including smoking and alcohol consumption were found to affect semen volume (Kunzle *et al.*, 2003). Mortimer *et al.*, (1982) found significant reduction in semen volume in polyzoospermia and azoospermia group participants. Minimum 1.5 mL of semen is required for smooth flow of the sperm and less than 1.5 mL volume the sperm will not buffer in vaginal acidity. Al-Ali *et al.*, (2014) found higher reduction of semen volume in obese and overweight oligozoospermia participants.

4.1.4 Sperm count

Table 4 shows that the mean sperm count was 87.1 million/mL (group 1), 54.4 million/mL (group 2), 46.7 million/mL (group 3), 8.8 million/mL (group 4) and 6.3 million/mL (group 5), respectively. It is found from **Figure 3** that the lower sperm count was seen in group 5 and the highest count was seen in group 1. The sperm count ranged from 39 to 160 million/mL (group 1), 21 to 97 million/mL (group 2), 26 to 99 million/mL (group 3), 5 to 12 million/mL (group 4) and 2 to 13 million/mL (group 5), respectively. Studies (Sharpe, 2012; Bonde *et al.*, 1998 and Attaman *et al.*, 2012) have shown that the sperm count plays an important role in pregnancy and many factors like pollution (Moline *et al.*, 2000) and environmental factors (Nordkap *et al.*, 2012) are responsible for low sperm count. Schlegel *et al.*, (1997) showed that the success rate of IVF is directly associated with sperm count. According to WHO (2010), less than 15 million/mL in a normal ejaculate is considered as low sperm count, but the study shows that around 2% of normozoospermia participants and 9% of oligozoospermia participants had sperm counts less than 10 million/mL (MacLeod *et al.*, 1951). A study shows that the sperm count was increased above 100 million/mL by treating with dexamethasone for 9 months (Nicopoullos *et al.*, 2003). In our study mean age of group 2–5 participants were above 35 years and a study shows that the sperm counts increased up to 34 years age and showing a decline phase immediately after 35 years (Stone *et al.*, 2013).

4.1.5 Sperm motility and Vitality

The motility of sperm was analyzed in all study participants and the results show that group 1 participants with 61.6%, followed by group 2 (41.2%), group 3 (22.3%), group 4 (24.5%) and group 5 (6.6%) of motile sperms respectively (**Figure 3**). It was found that there was no rapid motility observed in group 3 and 5 participants and observed 13.3% in group 1, followed by 2.5% in group 2 and 0.05% in group 4 respectively and (35.5%) group 1, (13.7%) group 2, (7.4%) group 3, (9.0%) group 4 and (2.0%) group 5 respectively with moderate motility. It was found that the least sluggish type of motility was seen in group 5 (4.1%) and highest sluggish type was seen in (25.0%) group 2 participants (**Figure 4**). Total sperm motility and three types of motility were showing statistically significant ($p<0.05$) among the study groups. From **Table 2**, it was found that the percentage of live sperms was 90.6% in group 1, 76.2% in group 2, 73.3% in group 3, 82.0% in group 4 and 43.2% in group 5 respectively. It was clear from **Figure 5** that group 1, 2 and 4 participants have normal live sperms percentage (>75%), but group 3 and 5 participants have lower than normal range. The mean dead sperm cells were 4.8%, 14.5%, 22.4%, 18.0% and 41.7% in groups 1–5, respectively. The maximum dead cells were found in group 5 participants and the minimum dead cells were found in group 1. Microscopic images of live and dead sperms among the different study groups are shown in **Plate 1**.

Internal and external changes in the body disturb the metabolism involved in head, neck and tail synthesis of sperm and thus alter the motility (Luconi, 2006). Appell *et al.*, (1977) states that body temperature influences the sperm motility and concluded that the motility of sperm was gradually decreased if the temperature was increased. Boyle *et al.*, (1993) conclude that reduction in sperm motility was the major reason for male infertility and, Barratt *et al.*, (1993) found that sperm velocity in the vagina is strongly associated with the conceive ability. Study shows that *in vivo* and *in vitro* fertility capacity of sperm was assessed mainly by sperm motility (Auger *et al.*, 1994). Elia *et al.*, (2010) concluded that the types of sperm motility include the rapid, moderate and sluggish which is a significant marker to assess the fertilizing capacity. Gonzales and Zapana (1992) states that sperm motility should be assessed after washing procedure, he concludes that participant was asthenozoospermia before washing, but its motility is improved after washing the semen. After removal of seminal plasma on the asthenospermia is reduced from 37.4 to 23.1 % and also found a reduction in sperm motility by addition of semen plasma in the washed sperm culture (Kanwar *et al.*, 1979). Khalili *et al.*, (1999) states that it is easy and useful to determine the live and dead sperm cells by vitality test even in asthenozoospermia.

4.1.6 Sperm Morphology

The percentage of normal sperm morphology was recorded in all study participants. It was found that only 9.3%, 1.9%, 4.5% and 1.8% of normal sperms was found in group 2 to 5. Normozoospermia group was found with maximum normal sperm (18.2%) and oligotetrazoospermia group was found with minimum normal sperm (1.8%). Microscopic images of sperm morphology among the different study group are shown in **Plate 2**. Roy *et al.*, (2001) concludes that cell morphology examination is the best tool to diagnose azoospermia. Low percentage of morphologically normal sperm cells was observed in groups 2 to 5 subjects when compared to group 1, which is highly correlated with the fertilizing capacity of the subjects. Similar supportive results were also found by Rogers *et al.*, (1983), Check and Bollendorf (1992) & Gopalakrishnan *et al.*, (1990). Kruger *et al.*, (1988) also reported that minimum 14% of normal morphology sperms required achieving fertilization. In our study group 2 to 5 have less than 14% of normal morphology sperm cells. Several studies have shown that sperm morphology is correlated with fertility capacity of the male partner (Dunphy *et al.*, 1989 and Bonde *et al.*, 1998). Uzunhisarcikli *et al.*, (2007) observed that exposures to heavy heat and chemical agents had high risk of increasing abnormal sperm morphology.

Table 4: Semen parameters of the study participants by group

Semen Analysis	Group 1 (n=9) (Mean±SEM)	Group 2 (n=16) (Mean±SEM)	Group 3 (n=13) (Mean±SEM)	Group 4 (n=10) (Mean±SEM)	Group 5 (n=12) (Mean±SEM)	p* value
Liquefaction (minutes)	28.5 ± 1.2	28.1 ± 1.6	28.3 ± 1.1	27.3 ± 1.6	24.8 ± 2.9	<0.05
pH	7.9 ± 0.13	7.8 ± 0.25	7.6 ± 0.33	7.8 ± 0.23	7.2 ± 0.62	0.53
Volume (mL)	4.1 ± 1.8	3.2 ± 1.6	3.0 ± 1.3	3.7 ± 1.9	2.8 ± 1.0	<0.05
Count (million/mL)	87.1 ± 36.6	54.4 ± 26.7	46.7 ± 20.6	8.8 ± 2.5	6.3 ± 4.4	<0.01
Motility (%)	65.5 ± 6.3	41.2 ± 21.7	22.3 ± 20.5	24.5 ± 13.0	6.6 ± 11.9	<0.01
Rapid (%)	13.3 ± 5.0	2.5 ± 3.6	0	0.05 ± 1.5	0	<0.01
Moderate (%)	35.5 ± 4.6	13.7 ± 8.2	7.4 ± 6.8	9.0 ± 5.1	2.0 ± 3.9	<0.01
Sluggish (%)	15.5 ± 5.2	25.0 ± 14.0	15.2 ± 14.1	14.5 ± 7.6	4.1 ± 8.2	<0.01
Live (%)	90.6 ± 2.8	76.2 ± 21.9	73.3 ± 18.0	82.0 ± 2.4	43.2 ± 22.9	<0.01
Dead (%)	4.8 ± 6.0	14.5 ± 10.4	22.4 ± 20.1	18.0 ± 2.4	41.7 ± 30.5	<0.01
Normal (%)	18.2 ± 4.8	9.3 ± 4.0	1.9 ± 0.7	4.5 ± 2.9	1.8 ± 0.7	<0.01

** $p < 0.05$ value denotes significance between groups*

Figure 2: Mean semen liquefaction time and pH of the study participants among the different groups

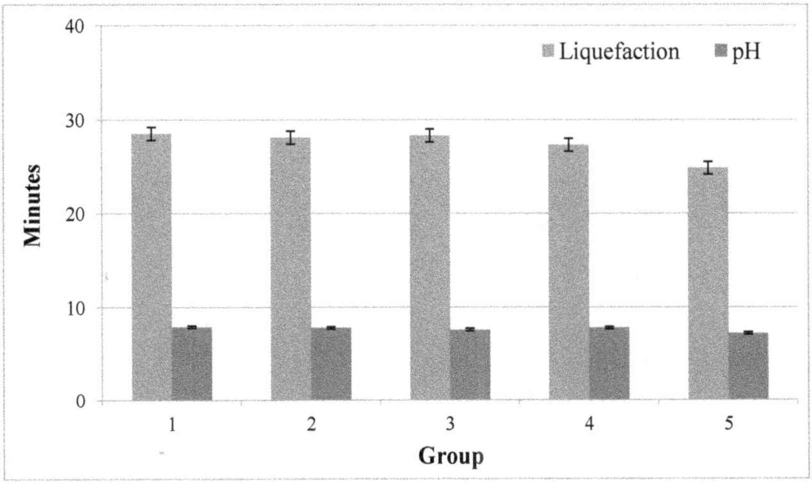

Figure 3: Mean semen volume, sperm count and motility of the study participants among the different groups

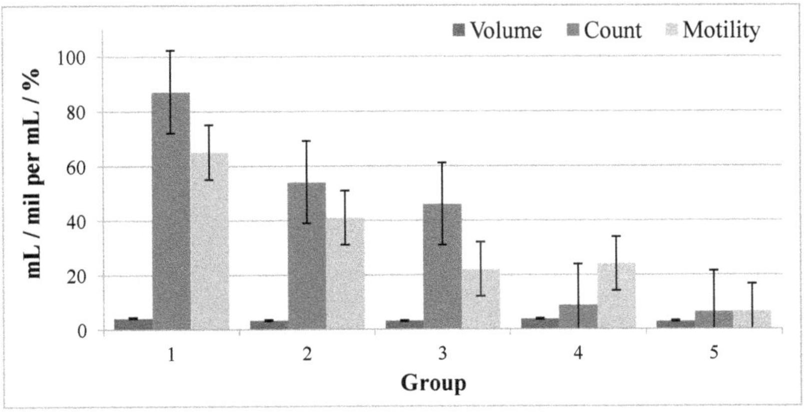

Figure 4: Mean percentage of types of sperm motility of the study participants among the different groups

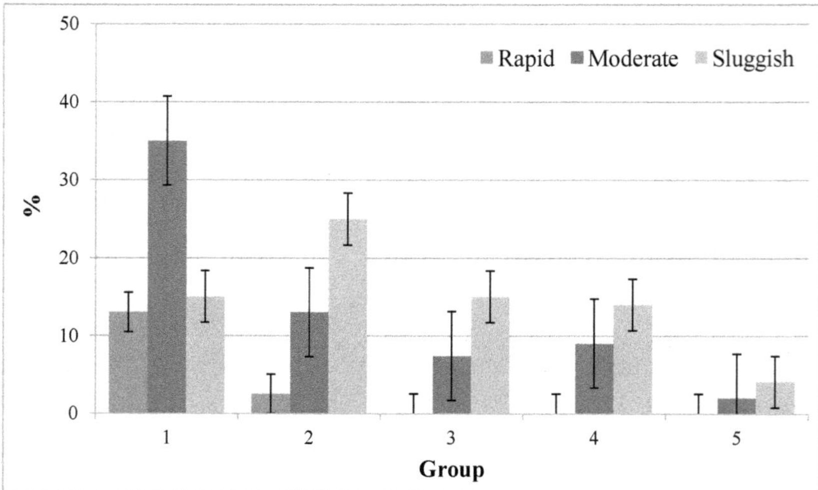

Figure 5: Mean percentage of live and dead sperm cells of the study participants among the different groups

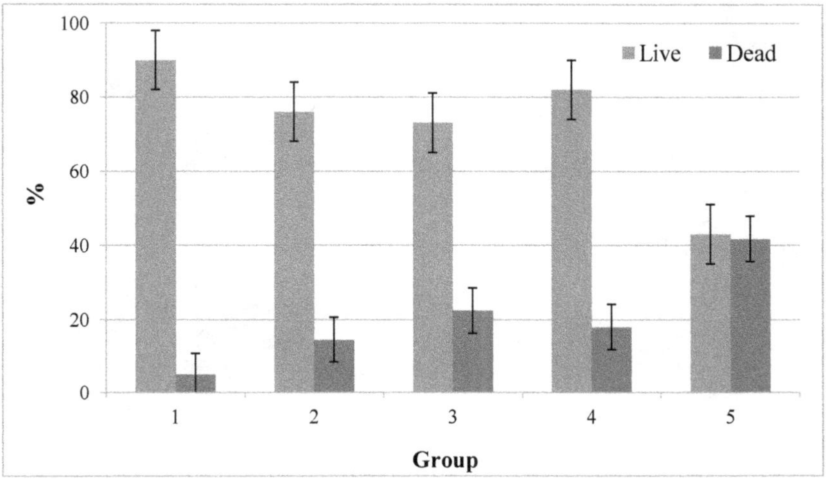

Figure 6: Mean percentage of normal sperm morphology of the study participants among the different groups

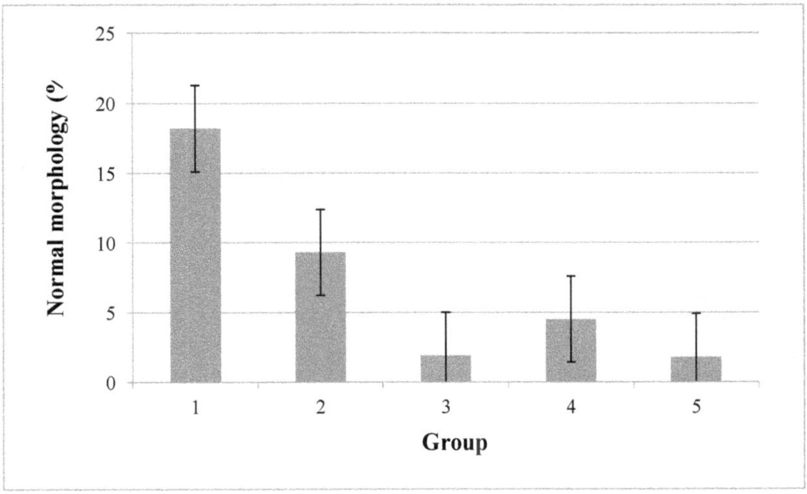

Plate 1: Live and dead sperms among the different study group

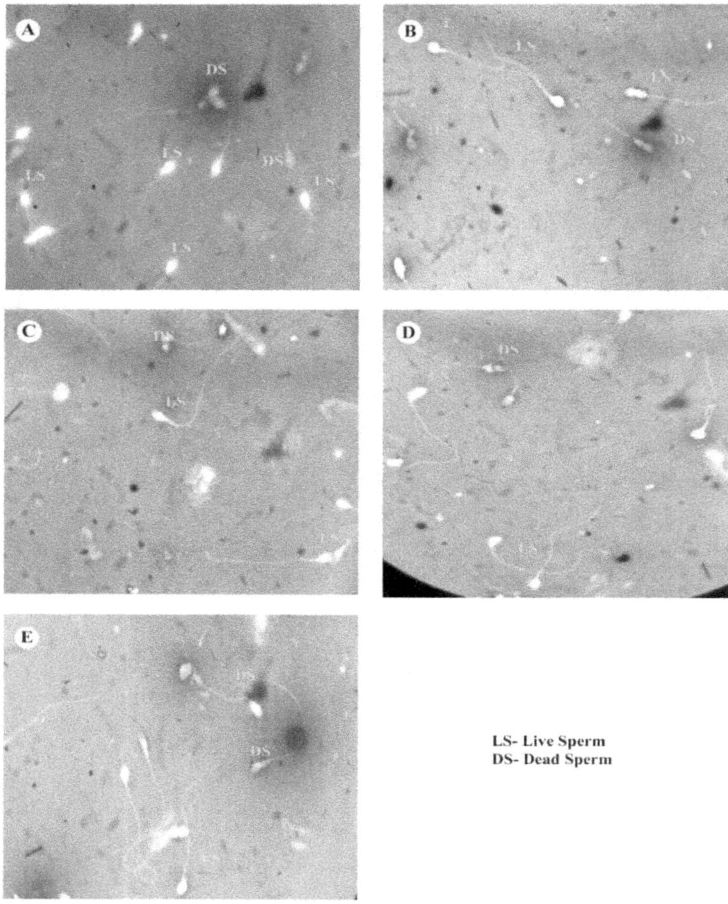

A. Normozoospermia, B. Asthenozoospermia, C. Asthenoteratozoospermia, D. Oligoasthenozoospermia
E. Oligoasthenoteratozoospermia

Plate 2: Morphology of sperms among the different study group

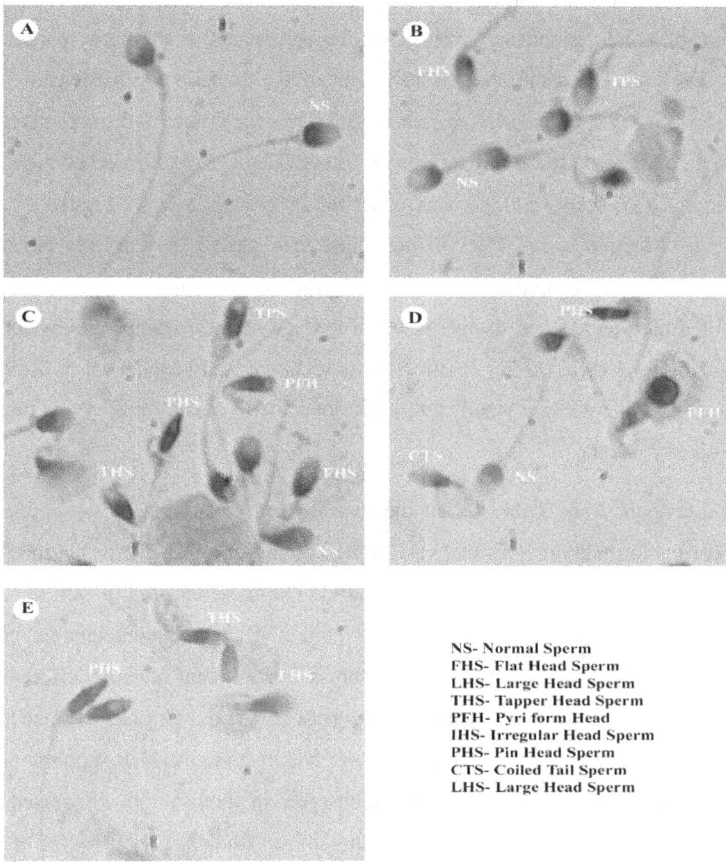

NS- Normal Sperm
FHS- Flat Head Sperm
LHS- Large Head Sperm
THS- Tapper Head Sperm
PFH- Pyri form Head
IHS- Irregular Head Sperm
PHS- Pin Head Sperm
CTS- Coiled Tail Sperm
LHS- Large Head Sperm

A. Normozoospermia, B. Asthenozoospermia, C. Asthenoteratozoospermia, D. Oligoasthenozoospermia E. Oligoasthenoteratozoospermia

4.2.1 Correlation between age and semen parameters

Anthropometric measurements were taken for all enrolled participants (**Table 5**). Association of semen parameters with metabolic parameters of the study participants are shown in **Table 6**. The result shows that the mean age of the study participants was 33.0 years, 37.1 years, 37.0 years, 34.3 years and 35.5 years for groups 1–5, respectively. It was found that among the study participants the lower age (33 years) was observed in group 1 and the higher age (37 years, $p<0.05$) was observed in groups 2 & 3 (**Figure 7**). A study conducted by Mathieu *et al.*, (1995), found that men aged <35 years are having higher fertility rates (52%) compared to men aged >35 years (25%). Another study shows that the majority of semen parameters decreased when the age of the participants increased which support our findings (Silea *et al.*, 2019). A cross sectional study conducted by Kumar *et al.*, (2017) found that there was a significant fall in total sperm count, motility and morphology after the age of 35 years.

It is evident from **Table 6** that the mean sperm count ($r= 0.03$, $p<0.05$) shows a negative correlation with age. Similar results were found on mean sperm motility ($r= 0.60$, $p<0.05$) and sperm morphology ($r= 0.62$, $p<0.05$). The minimum fall in semen parameters was observed at a younger age and the maximum fall in all semen parameters was noted after 35 years. Our study clearly shows that age shows a significant negative effect on semen parameters. A study compared the semen quality between 30 and 50 years old men and found decrease in count, motility and volume when age was increased which supports our results (Kidd *et al.*, 2001). Similar findings were also observed in another study conducted in 22–80 years old men (Eskenazi *et al.*, 2003). Many other studies also observed a negative correlation between age and semen parameters (Girsh *et al.*, 2008 & Klonoff-Cohen and Natarajan, 2004). Studies conducted by Rolf *et al.*, (1996) observed decline in sperm counts with aging and our study also revealed similar findings. Several other studies found similar results with age and sperm count (Winkle *et al.*, 2009; Moskovtsev *et al.*, 2009 and Stone *et al.*, 2013). In contrast to our findings a Spain study examined in 22 thousand infertile males found significant increase in sperm count with age (Andolz *et al.*, 1999). Some other authors did not observe any correlation between age and semen parameters (Berling and Wolner-Hanssen, 1997 & Spandorfer *et al.*, 1998). In our study the sperm motility decreased with age and similar findings was observed by Auger *et al.*, 1995; Sloter *et al.*, 2006 and Fisch *et al.*, 1996. Apart from count and motility, the morphology of sperm declines with increase in age and similar findings was reported by Mukhopadhyay *et al.*, 2010; Silva *et al.*, 2012 and

Braga *et al*, 2011, but other studies did not find any correlation between age and sperm morphology (Kidd *et al*., 2001; Brahem *et al*., 2011; Dain *et al*., 2011 and Nijs *et al*., 2011).

4.2.2 Correlation between bodyweight and BMI with semen parameters

The result of **Table 5** shows that the mean body weight of study participants was 73.6 Kg, 84.8 Kg, 95.7 Kg, 93.6 Kg and 84.6 Kg for groups 1–5, respectively. Among the study groups, the participants in group 3 are showing higher body weight (95.7 Kg, $p<0.05$) when compare to other groups of participants. **Figure 9** shows the graphical representation of mean BMI of study participants. The mean BMI was 23.2 Kg/m^2, 27.7 Kg/m^2, 30.8 Kg/m^2, 28.6 Kg/m^2 and 28.2 Kg/m^2 for groups 1–5, respectively. It is evident from **Table 5** that the highest BMI was observed in group 3 participants (30.8 Kg/m^2) which means that most of the participants were overweight and the lowest BMI was observed in group 1 (23.2 Kg/m^2) with normal BMI.

Male obesity is one of the risk factors for abnormal semen parameters. Similar to our findings, a cross sectional study shows that men with BMI >30 have poor semen quality when compared to men with normal BMI (Shayeb *et al*., 2011). Another study results show that the sperm concentration (25.7 million/mL) was lower in men with BMI 25–29 Kg/m^2 when compared to normal BMI males (Alahmar *et al*., 2018). The incidence of oligozoospermia (9.2% and 15.6%) was found higher in overweight and obese participants when compared to normal (5.3%) BMI group (Hammoud *et al*., 2008).

The data from **Figure 10** shows that the mean sperm count ($r= -0.43$, $p<0.05$; $r= -0.31$, $p<0.05$) was found to have a negative correlation with body weight and BMI respectively. Similar trend was noticed for sperm motility (weight: $r= -0.23$, $p<0.05$; BMI: $r= -0.20$, $p<0.05$) and morphology (weight: $r= -0.10$, $p<0.05$; BMI: $r= -0.89$, $p<0.05$) (**Figure 11**). Numerous studies found a relationship between body weight, BMI and semen parameters. Studies conducted by Chavarro *et al*., 2010; Kort *et al*., 2006; Sekhavat and Moein, 2010; Hakonsen *et al*., 2011 and Paasch *et al*., 2010 observed negative correlation between BMI and sperm count, which support our findings, but MacDonald *et al*., (2010) reported a negative correlation only in infertile group but not in fertile group. Studies show that significant negative correlation exists between BMI and sperm motility (Hofny *et al*., 2010 and Fejes *et al*., 2006), but Hammoud *et al*., (2008b) reported significant improvement in sperm motility with increased BMI. Jensen *et al*., (2004) not found any association between BMI and sperm motility. The sperm morphology of the study subjects also shows a negative correlation with BMI. Hajshafiha *et al*., (2013) reported that higher BMI is one of the risk factors for increasing the prevalence of oligozoospermia. Hammoud *et al*., (2008b) observed high level of abnormal morphology sperms in obesity group. Higher level of oestradiol lead to a reduction in testosterone concentration in obese men results in abnormal morphology (Hammiche *et al*., 2012). Few studies reported that there is no relationship between semen parameters and BMI (Duits *et al*., 2010; Eskandar *et al*., 2012 and Mormandi *et al*., 2013). A study conducted by Qin *et al*., (2007) and Jensen *et al*., (2004) reported poor semen quality in underweight compared to normal and overweight group. A study conducted by Rufus *et al*., (2018) did not find any significant differences in semen quality between normal BMI and elevated BMI group. Studies observed low pregnancy in obese men undergoing ART (Bakos *et al*., 2011 and Hinz *et al*., 2010). Few studies conclude that obese men have higher chance to get an obese child like father (Danielzik *et al*., 2002 and Li, *et al*., 2009). Studies reported that inducing obesity in male by feeding a high fat diet shows a reduction in sperm motility and normal morphology (Palmer *et al*., 2012 and Fernandez *et al*., 2011).

4.2.3 Correlation between blood pressure and semen parameters

Mean systolic blood pressure was 122.0 mmHg, 138.8 mmHg, 145.0 mmHg, 130.0 mmHg and 133.6 mmHg for groups 1–5, respectively and diastolic blood pressure was 77.7 mmHg, 80.1 mmHg, 84.0 mmHg, 89.5 mmHg and 92.0 mmHg from the groups 1–5, respectively. Both systolic and diastolic blood pressures were observed to be high in all other groups when compared to group 1 (**Figure 12**).

Figures 13 & **14** show that mean sperm count (Sys: $r = -0.58$, $p<0.05$; Dia: $r = -0.54$; $p<0.05$), sperm motility (Sys: $r = -0.73$, $p<0.05$; Dia: $r = -0.43$; $p<0.05$); and morphology (Sys: $r = -0.55$, $p<0.05$; Dia: $r = -0.48$; $p<0.05$) show significant negative correlation with blood pressure. Studies show that the incidence of male infertility gradually increased in hypertensive male (Zhao *et al*., 2010 and Azu, 2015). Many studies found the significant relationship between blood pressure and semen quality (Phillips *et al*., 1993 and Fogari *et al*., 2002). More than one semen abnormalities was observed in hypertensive men compared to normal group (Eisenberg *et al*., 2015 and Guo *et al*., 2015). Svartberg *et al*., (2004) demonstrated a negative association between systolic blood pressure and total testosterone concentration. Studies conducted by Suzuki *et al*., (1988), Andersen *et al*., (1998) and Koshida *et al*., (1998) show that there is no significant reduction in testosterone levels after treating with hypertensive agents. Guo *et al*., (2017) concluded that various hypertensive medications lead to poor semen quality. Cazzaniga *et al*., (2020) did not find any significant difference in semen parameters between oligozoospermia, asthenozoospermia and teratozoospermia compared to normal group. Akinyemi *et al*., (2015) found significant improvement in semen parameters in hypertensive rat after ginger and turmeric supplementation. Higher prevalence rate of erectile dysfunction (ED) was observed in hypertensive males compared to normal (Viigimaa *et al*., 2014).

Table 5: Anthropometric profiles of the study participants by group

Variables	Group 1 (n=9) (Mean ± SEM)	Group 2 (n=16) (Mean ± SEM)	Group 3 (n=13) (Mean ± SEM)	Group 4 (n=10) (Mean ± SEM)	Group 5 (n=12) (Mean ± SEM)	p* value
Age (Years)	33.0 ± 3.4	37.1 ± 7.2	37.0 ± 6.4	34.3 ± 5.8	35.5 ± 4.8	<0.05
Weight (Kg)	73.6 ± 8.0	84.8 ± 15.4	95.7 ± 9.2	93.6 ±1 3.8	84.6 ± 5.9	<0.05
BMI (Kg/m^2)	23.2 ± 4.0	27.7 ± 5.0	30.8 ± 2.8	28.6 ± 4.4	28.2 ± 2.3	<0.01
BP-SYS (mmHg)	122.0 ± 7.0	138.8 ± 5.4	145.0 ± 10.9	130.5 ± 9.5	133.6 ± 9.3	<0.05
BP-DIA (mmHg)	77.7 ± 4.4	80.1 ± 5.1	84.0 ± 11.0	89.5 ± 8.9	92.0 ± 6.0	<0.05

*p < *0.05 value denotes significance between groups*

Table 6: Association of semen parameters with metabolic parameters of the study participants

Variables	Sperm count		Sperm Motility		Sperm Morphology	
	Pearson correlation	p value	Pearson correlation	p value	Pearson correlation	p value
Age (Years)	–0.33	<0.05	–0.60	<0.05	–0.62	<0.05
Weight (Kg)	–0.43	<0.05	–0.23	<0.05	–0.10	<0.05
BMI (Kg/m^2)	–0.31	<0.05	–0.20	<0.05	–0.89	<0.05
Systolic (mmHg)	–0.58	0.13	–0.73	0.15	–0.55	0.14
Diastolic (mmHg)	–0.54	0.19	–0.43	0.72	–0.48	0.21

Figure 7: Mean age of study participants among the different groups

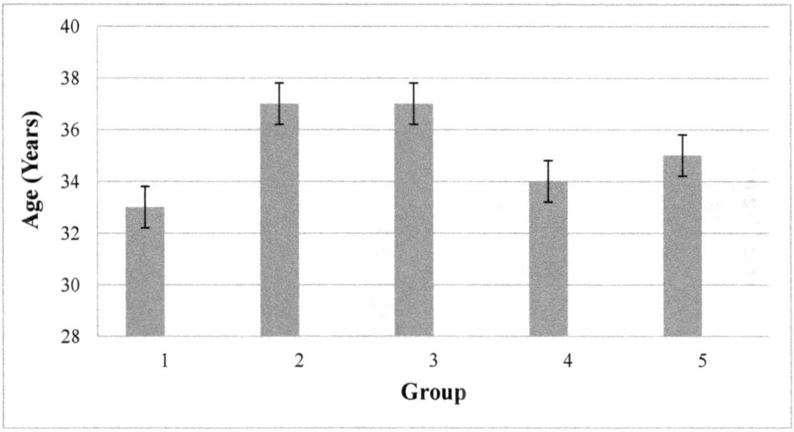

Figure 8: Scatter plots and linear regression lines of age and semen parameters of the study participants

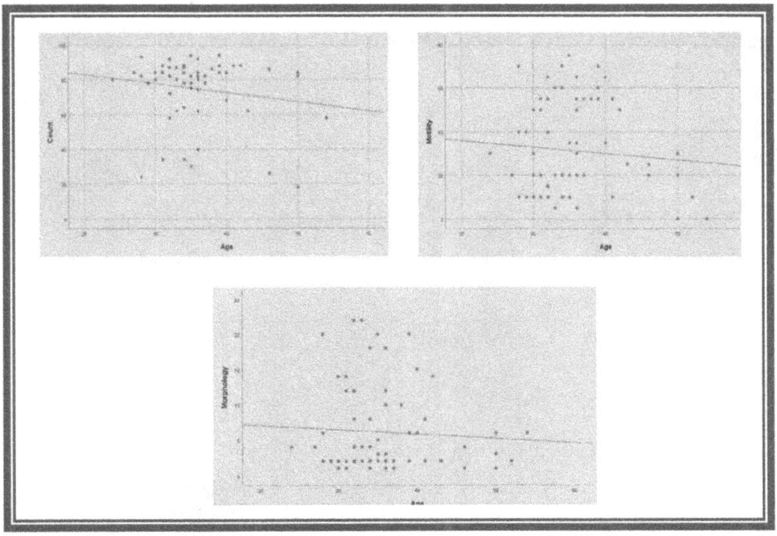

Figure 9: Mean body weight and BMI of study participants among the different groups

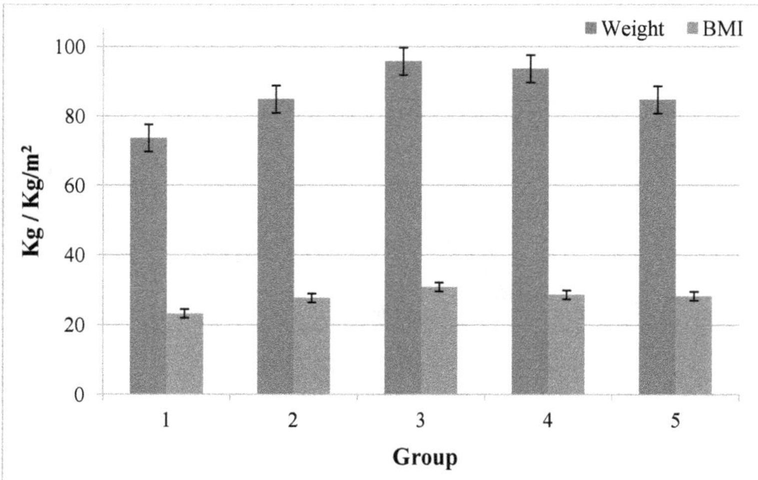

Figure 10: Scatter plots and linear regression lines of body weight and semen parameters of the study participants

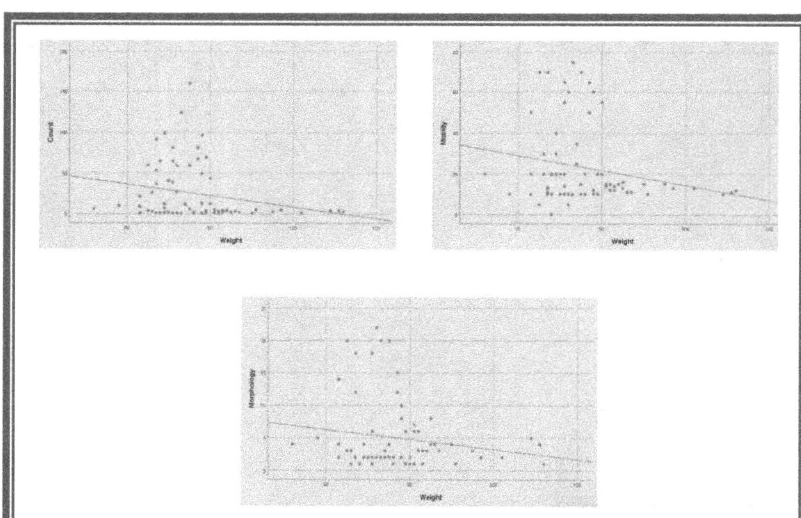

Figure 11: Scatter plots and linear regression lines of BMI and semen parameters of the study participants

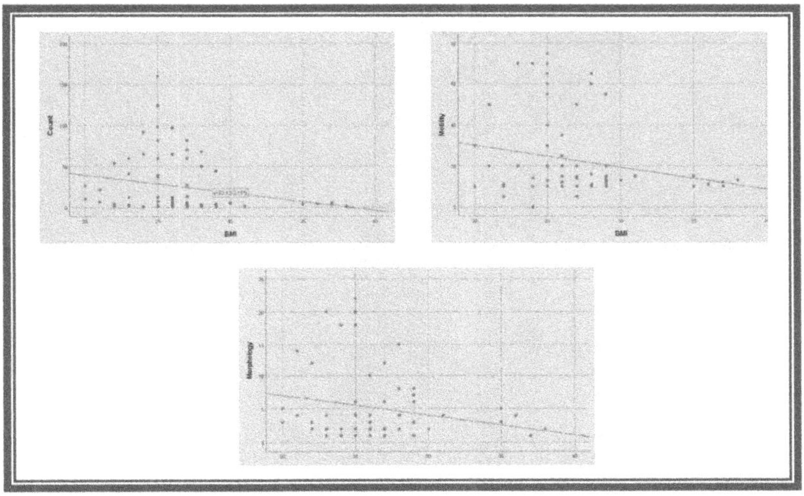

Figure 12: Mean systolic and diastolic blood pressures of study participants among the different groups

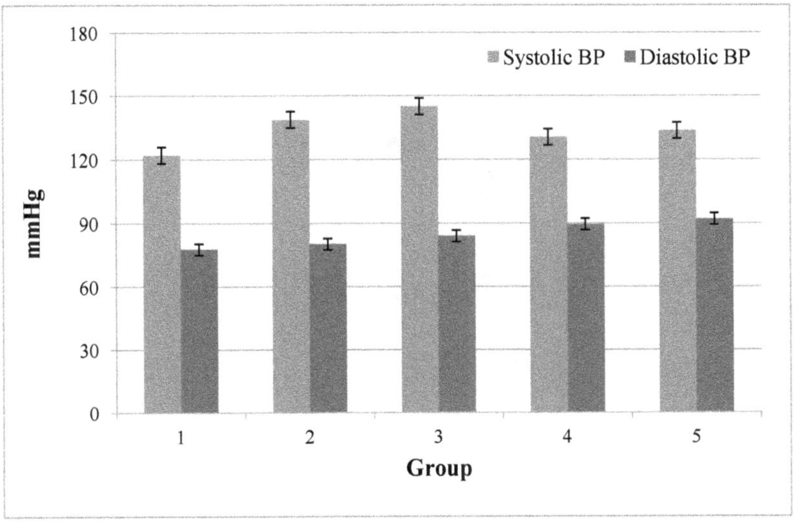

Figure 13: Scatter plots and linear regression lines of systolic blood pressure and semen parameters of the study participants

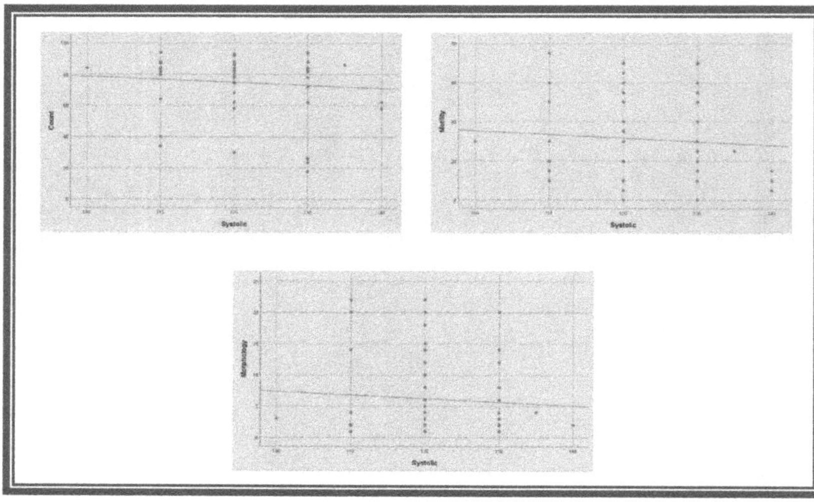

Figure 14: Scatter plots and linear regression lines of diastolic blood pressure and semen parameters of the study participants

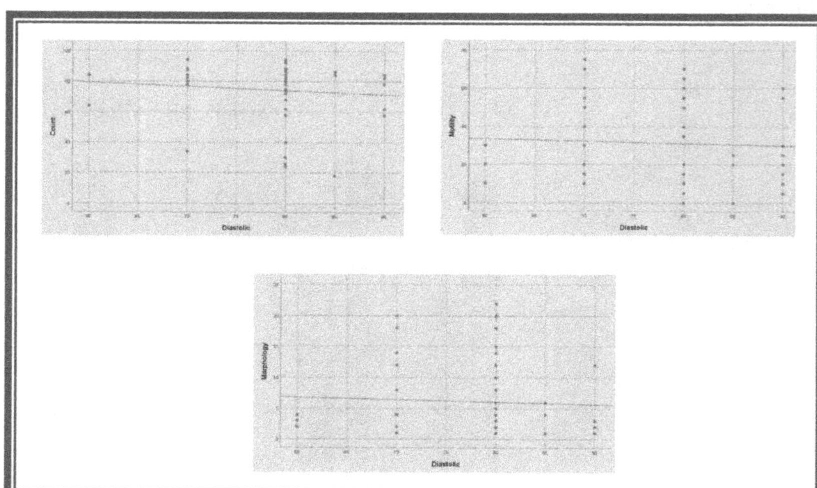

4.3 Trace metals profile of the study groups

4.3.1 Correlation between calcium and semen parameters

The trace metal profile of the participants is shown in **Table 7** and the Pearson correlation between trace metal and semen parameters is shown in **Table 8**. It was found that the mean calcium concentration in seminal plasma was observed as 10.6 mg/dL, 15.5 mg/dL and 18.6 mg/dL for groups 1–3, respectively, but the groups 4 and 5 show slightly higher concentration (22.6 mg/dL and 24.2 mg/dL). There is a significant difference in calcium concentration among groups 1–5. **Figure 16** shows that mean sperm count ($r = 0.67$, $p<0.05$), sperm motility ($r = 0.79$, $p<0.05$) and morphology ($r = 0.45$; $p<0.05$) show a significant positive correlation with calcium level.

Among trace metal Calcium is widely studied element in human semen (Jensen *et al.*, 2016). And many studies reported the level of calcium in human semen (Skandhan *et al.*, 1978a and Valsa *et al.*, 1994 & 2012). Studies showed the role of calcium ions in sperm motility (Darszon *et al.*, 2005 and Fakih *et al.*, 1986), fertilization (Yanagimachi, 1981 & Yanagimachi and Usai, 1974). Many semen parameters include motility, acrosome synthesis was calcium dependent and showed poor semen quality by calcium deficiency (Harchegani *et al.*, 2019). Calcium plays as intercellular signaling molecule to fertilize the oocyte in the female reproductive track (Valsa *et al.*, 2015). Prostate gland is the richest source of calcium ions (Valsa *et al.*, 2016). Several studies have reported the association between seminal calcium level and male infertility (Darszon *et al.*, 2011 and Hommonai *et al.*, 1978). Similar to our results, the studies conducted by Prien *et al.*, (1990) and Wong *et al.*, (2001) found lower concentration of calcium with low sperm motility in infertile subjects compared to normal group. A study shows a positive correlation between fertility and seminal plasma calcium concentration (Logoglu *et al.*, 1997) and result showed a significant reduction in seminal plasma Calcium level in normozoospermic infertile compared with the fertile male. Studies conducted by Nishida *et al.*, (1996), found that fertilizing capacity of sperm increased when *in vitro* exposure to low Ca concentration culture medium. Owen *et al.*, (2005) & Lindholmer and Eliasson (1974) found a positive relationship between calcium and semen parameters which supports our results.

4.3.2 Correlation between magnesium and semen parameters

Table 7 and **Figure 15** gives a clear picture on the mean magnesium concentration in seminal plasma of the study participants and it was found to be 2.2 mg/dL (Group 1); 2.9 mg/dL (Group 2); 5.4 mg/dL (Group 3); 4.3 mg/dL (Group 4) and 8.5 mg/dL (Group 5) of magnesium. There is a statistically significant difference in magnesium concentration among the study groups. The results of Pearson correlation shows that mean sperm count ($r= 0.23$, $p<0.05$), sperm motility ($r= 0.48$, $p<0.05$); and morphology ($r= 0.61$; $p<0.05$) show significant positive correlation with magnesium level (**Figure 17**).

A study conducted in Nigeria showed abnormal level of magnesium in infertile groups compared with fertile group (Bassey *et al.*, 2013), which supports our findings, but Saglam *et al.*, (2015) reported that there is no significant difference in magnesium concentration between fertile and infertile men. Different studies show various conclusions, but the exact role of magnesium in semen is unclear. Magnesium level observed to have a negative correlation with seminal parameters (Banjoko, 2013) also supports our findings. Deger and Akkus (1988) reported that magnesium level was nearly 11.9 mg/dL in fertile and 6.9 mg/dL in infertile subjects. Studies show that magnesium was used as a marker for prostate infection (Papadimas *et al.*, 1983) and also observed magnesium deficiency associated with high thromboxane level that lead to premature ejaculation (Omu *et al.*, 2001). According to Morisawa (1982), the magnesium acts as cofactor for enzymes involved in sperm motility. Studies show that magnesium concentration shows a positive effect on sperm motility (Kiss, 1983 and Kovacsne-Gaal, 1994). Viski *et al.*, (1995) found 30–35% damaged sperms in oligozoospermic and asthenozoospermic men compared to normal group and found positive relationship between magnesium and other semen parameters. Studies conducted in rat shows that magnesium sulphate shows improvement in semen parameters (Asghari *et al.*, 2016). Wong *et al.*, (2001) shows a strong correlation between magnesium and with sperm count but not on sperm motility which support our findings. Zavaczki *et al.*, (2003) found significant improvement in sperm count, motility and viability in infertile men after treating magnesium orotate (3000 mg/day) for 90 days.

4.3.3 Correlation between zinc and semen parameters

One of the important trace metals is zinc, which is required for normal spermatogenesis and a decreased level of zinc shows impact on testicular function in males (Ali *et al.*, 2005). The mean zinc level was 6.3 mg/dL, 4.1 mg/dL, 2.0 mg/dL, 1.6 mg/dL and

1.4 mg/dL for groups 1–5, respectively (**Figure 15**). The lowest level was observed in group 5 participants and the highest level was observed significantly ($p<0.05$) for group 1 participants. Graphical presentation of Pearson correlation shows that the mean sperm count ($r= 0.60$, $p<0.05$), sperm motility ($r= 0.71$, $p<0.05$); and morphology ($r= 0.31$; $p<0.05$) show significant positive correlation with zinc level (**Figure 18**).

Higher concentration of zinc was observed at reproductive track (Bedwal and Bahuguna, 1994) and found there are no changes in zinc concentration before and after vasectomy (Parrish *et al.*, 1987). An animal study shows that lower level of zinc lead to decreasing testosterone level (Omu *et al.*, 2015). In our study, seminal zinc levels were higher in normozoospermia compared to other groups, and similar results were found by Camejo *et al.*, 2011; Chia *et al.*, 2000 and Atig *et al.*, 2012. The quality of semen was improved and also found a reduction in anti-sperm antibodies in asthenozoospermia group of zinc supplementation (Omu *et al.*, 1998 and Raigani *et al.*, 2014). Few studies found that zinc concentration was lower in infertile group compared to normal group (Zheng *et al.*, 2012; Liao *et al.*, 2008 and Zhang *et al.*, 2003) which support our findings but few studies reported that there is no significance difference in zinc concentration between infertile and fertile group (Colagar *et al.*, 2009 and Fuse *et al.*, 1999). One study concludes that the zinc concentration was significantly higher in the abnormal group compared to the normal group (Akinloye *et al.*, 2011). Shquirat *et al.*, 2013 found a low concentration of zinc and poor semen quality in infertile men compared to fertile group. Wong *et al.*, (2001), found higher concentration of zinc in both seminal plasma and serum in fertile compared to fertile group. Wroblewska *et al.*, (2011) and Camejo *et al.*, (2011) reported that there was no statistically significant difference in zinc level between varicocele and normozoospermia. Yuyan *et al.*, (2008) observed low zinc level in serum of asthenozoospermia group.

4.3.4 Correlation between sodium and potassium and semen parameters

Similar to other body cells, normal sperm cells also have sodium and potassium pump (Quinn and White, 1967). Seminal plasma is a nutrient medium for sperm function, metabolism, survival and transport in female track. Na and K serve to maintain the osmotic balance, which play as cofactors for many important enzymes. Studies show that abnormal concentration of Na and K leads to reproductive disorder (Barrier-Battut *et al.*, 2002 and Massanyi *et al.*, 2004).

The mean Na level was 148.3 mEq/L, 139.4 mEq/L, 132.0 mEq/L, 128.8 mEq/L and 120.2 mEq/L in groups 1–5, respectively. There are no significant differences in Na level among the study groups. With regard to K, the mean level was 5.0, 13.2, 22.8, 22.4 and 22.6 mEq/L (**Figure 19**). **Figures 20 & 21** show that the mean sperm count (Na: $r = -0.19$, $p > 0.05$; K: $r = -0.47$, $p < 0.05$), sperm motility (Na: $r = -0.35$, $p < 0.05$; K: $r = -0.16$, $p > 0.05$) and sperm morphology (Na: $r = -0.14$, $p > 0.05$; K: $r = -0.15$, $p > 0.05$) show a week positive correlation with sodium and potassium ions.

Kanwal *et al.*, (2000) and Abdel-Rahman *et al.*, (2000) also observed similar results in bull and found a negative correlation with semen volume and semen parameters. Studies conducted by Gusani *et al.*, (1988); Sheth and Rao (1962) & Mann (1964) found a positive correlation between sodium and sperm motility and also found negative correlation between potassium and sperm motility in oligoasthenozoospermia. Hamad *et al.*, (2014) found significant differences in viscosity, motility, in normal and infertile men and also observed a significant decrease in K in the infertile group. N'Guessan *et al.*, (2016) reported no significant difference in sodium and potassium concentration in seminal plasma between normozoospermic and azoospermic groups. Adekunbi *et al.*, (2016) found that sperm function was affected by increasing the sodium and potassium level in the blood by consuming high salt diet. Skandhan and Mazumdar, (1981a) observed normal sperm motility when the sodium and potassium concentration was within reference range and found alternation in sperm motility when the sodium and potassium concentration was changed.

4.3.5 Correlation between copper and semen parameters

In the present study, seminal plasma copper concentration was compared among 5 groups. The mean copper concentration was 81.0 µg/L, 142.0 µg/L, 154.0 µg/L, 149.0 µg/L and 167.0 µg/L in groups 1–5, respectively. **Figure 22** shows that seminal plasma copper concentration was higher ($p < 0.05$) in groups 4 & 5 compared to normal group 1. Scatter plots shows that the mean sperm count ($r = 0.74$, $p < 0.05$), sperm motility ($r = 0.35$, $p > 0.05$), and sperm morphology ($r = 0.12$, $p > 0.05$) are positively associated with copper concentration. The result shows that copper level was significantly associated with sperm count but not with sperm motility and sperm morphology (**Figure 23**).

A study conducted by Wong *et al.*, (2001) shows a weak positive correlation between motility and copper concentration, as in our case. In another study positive correlation was found with count, motility and morphology when copper concentration was within range, but shows a negative correlation in abnormal concentration (Jockenhovel *et al.*, 1990), which supports our results that abnormal groups show higher concentration compared to the normal group. Aydemir *et al.*, (2006) also observed higher concentration of copper in blood serum and seminal plasma in the infertile group compared to normal fertile group. Many other studies conducted by various researchers show that higher concentration of copper shows adverse effects in semen quality (Katayose *et al.*, 2004 and Salsabili *et al.*, 2009), but studies by Yuyan *et al.*, (2008) concludes that there is no significant effect of higher or low seminal plasma copper concentration with semen quality. In our study, we observed higher concentration of copper in abnormal groups compared to normal groups. Similarly Maryam Eidi *et al.*, (2010) reported that higher copper concentration in oligozoospermic, asthenozoospermic and azoospermic groups compared to normal group. Consuming a diet with a higher concentration of copper shows an adverse effect on male and female reproductive organs (Katayose *et al.*, 2004 and Jockenhovel *et al.*, 1990). Ogorek *et al.*, (2017) reported higher or lower concentration of copper shows negative impact on spermatogenesis. Kasperczyk *et al.*, (2016) reported that there is no significant difference in volume, pH, count, motility and morphology of sperm between copper exposure and non-exposure group.

4.3.6 Correlation between selenium and semen parameters

Selenium act as cofactor for many enzymes and helps to protect cells. Higher concentration was observed in testis, seminal vesicles and prostate. **Figure 22** shows that the selenium concentration was found as 178.2 µg/L (Group 1), 77.6 µg/L (Group 2), 52.2 µg/L (Group 3), 56.4 µg/L (Group 4) and 47.3 µg/L (Group 5). **Figure 24** shows that the mean sperm count ($r = 0.73$, $p < 0.05$), sperm motility ($r = 0.65$, $p < 0.05$), and sperm morphology ($r = 0.16$, $p > 0.05$) shows a positive correlation with seminal plasma selenium level. From **Table 7**, it was clear that lower ($p < 0.05$) selenium concentration was observed in abnormal group 2–5 compared to the normal group 1.

Hurst *et al.*, (1999) reported that infertile males had significantly lower seminal plasma selenium level compared to fertile group, which supports our findings. Studies conducted by Camejo *et al.*, (2011); Eroglu *et al.*, (2014) and Oldereid *et al.*, (1998) found a positive relationship between seminal plasma selenium concentration and sperm count, but Atig *et al.*, (2012) and Li *et al.*, (2012) observed negative relationship with selenium concentration. A study was observed higher selenium level in blood serum and seminal plasma after oral administration (100–300 mcg/day), but it not shown any changes in semen parameters in abnormal group (Scott *et al.*, 1998) and also in normal group males (Hawkes *et al.*, 2009). In contrast, the study observed improvement in semen parameters and hormone profiles in infertile males after consuming selenium capsules 50 μg/day once at night (Morbat *et al.*, 2018). In another study examine the combination of selenium and vitamins A, C and E pills for three months and found significant improvement in sperm motility (Scott *et al.*, 1998) and selenium protect sperm DNA from oxidation thus enhance the count and motility (Lerda, 1992). Krsnjavi *et al.*, (1992) reported lower level of selenium in seminal plasma and blood in oligozoospermia and azoospermia group compared to control group. Logistic regression models of this study shows that higher selenium level was found in oilgospermia than azoospermia. A Canadian study shows that the significant improvement in motility, viability and morphology after treated infertile patients with 100 μg of selenium daily (Vezina *et al.*, 1996). Other studies also show the positive correlation with selenium and semen parameters (Akinloye *et al.*, 2005 and Lerda, 1992).

4.3.7 Correlation between chromium and semen parameters

Chromium act as cofactor for many enzymes implicated in spermatogenesis, lower and higher concentration shows poor semen quality in humans (Meeker *et al.*, 2008). Chromium concentration was assessed on seminal plasma and the results show that 2.2 μg/dL, 4.2 μg/dL, 4.9 μg/dL, 4.6 μg/dL and 5.8 μg/dL in groups 1–5, respectively. It was found that chromium concentration was observed high ($p<0.05$) in the abnormal group when compared to normal group 1 (**Figure 25**). Data on Pearson coefficient correlation shows that the mean sperm count ($r= -0.57$, $p<0.05$), sperm motility ($r= -0.36$, $p<0.05$), and sperm morphology ($r= -0.28$, $p<0.05$) was negatively correlated with chromium level in seminal plasma (**Figure 26**).

Studies carried out by Skandhan *et al.*, (2005) and Umeyama *et al.*, (1986) also found similar results about semen parameters and chromium concentration in oilgozoospermia and normozoospermia groups. Few experimental studies found that abnormal level of chromium reduces sperm count and motility by causing testicular atrophy (Saxena *et al.*, 1990 and Ernst, 1990). Studies found that occupational exposure group shows adverse effects on semen quality when compared to non-occupational exposure group (Kumar *et al.*, 2005 and Li *et al.*, 2001). Li *et al.*, (1999) found damaged seminiferous tubules, reduction in spermatogenesis and a higher prevalence rate of teratozoospermia in subject exposure to certain level of chromium. Yan *et al*., (2014) found the higher seminal plasma chromium level and abnormal semen parameters in participants resident in environmental polluted site in China compared with control group. Danadevi *et al*., (2003) conducted a study in welding workers in south India and found significant positive correlation between chromium level and semen abnormalities in welding workers compared to control group. Similar study conducted by Kumar *et al*., (2005) and Meeker *et al.,* (2008), found a higher percentage of abnormal sperm morphology in occupational exposure workers compares to the normal group. Elhafeez *et al*., (2019) observed testicular damage in male albino rats treated with Cr (1.25 mg/Kg) for 65 days.

4.3.8 Correlation between lead and semen parameters

Role of lead and semen parameter is not clear, as this may involve in any metabolic pathway. **Figure 25** shows that the mean lead concentration in seminal plasma was 19.34 μg/L, 40.24 μg/L, 156.34 μg/L, 161.24 μg/L and 175.4 μg/L in groups 1–5, respectively. From the scatter plot shows that the mean sperm count ($r = -0.71$, $p<0.05$), sperm motility ($r = -0.20$, $p>0.05$), and sperm morphology ($r = -0.57$, $p<0.05$) shows a negative correlation with seminal lead level (**Figure 27**).

It is evident from **Table 7** that higher ($p<0.05$) concentration of lead in seminal plasma was observed in the abnormal group 2–5 when compared to normal group 1. Pant *et al*., (2015) found a negative correlation with seminal plasma lead and semen parameters which support our findings. The author also concludes that smoking is the main exposure of lead in the infertile group. Similar to our findings, Telisman *et al*., (2000) found a negative correlation between seminal plasma lead and count ($r = -0.17$, $p<0.05$), motility ($r = -0.17$, $p<0.05$) and morphology ($r = 0.20$, $p<0.05$).

Studies shows that the higher lead concentration shows negative impact on semen parameters include count, motility and morphology in occupational exposure group (Alexander *et al*., 1996 & 1998 and Lahdetie, 1995). Studies show that lead directly influence the sperm motility (Naha *et al*., 2005 and Viskum *et al*., 1999), viability (Hernandez-Ochoa *et al*., 2005), reduction in maturity of sperm cells (Wildt *et al*., 1983), low success rate in ART (Benoff *et al*., 2003), decrease the percentage of sperm reaching ova (Chowdhuri *et al*., 2001), unable to penetrate the oocyte (Johansson, 1989), loss of embryos after implantations (Al-Hakkak *et al*., 1988), destruction in androgen binding (Goyer, 2001), decrease the FSH production (Wiebe *et al*., 1983), affect the function of Sertoli cell (Batarseh *et al*., 1986) and decrease activity of testicular oxidizing enzymes (Winder, 1989). Debnath *et al.*, (2010) reported no significant correlation in seminal plasma and blood lead concentration between infertile and fertile males. Authors also conclude that the main reason that both groups were from the same environment.

Table 7: Concentration of trace metals in the seminal plasma of the study participants

Trace metals	Group 1 (n=9) (Mean ± SEM)	Group 2 (n=16) (Mean ± SEM)	Group 3 (n=13) (Mean ± SEM)	Group 4 (n=10) (Mean ± SEM)	Group 5 (n=12) (Mean ± SEM)	p* value
Ca (mg/dL)	10.6 ± 0.01	15.5 ± 0.08	18.6 ± 0.05	22.6 ± 0.06	24.2 ± 0.06	<0.05
Mg (mEq/L)	2.2 ± 0.01	2.9 ± 0.07	5.4 ± 0.06	4.3 ± 0.09	8.5 ± 0.10	0.09
Zn (mg/dL)	6.3 ± 0.03	4.1 ± 0.09	2.0 ± 0.06	1.6 ± 0.10	1.4 ± 0.01	<0.05
Na (mEq/L)	148.3 ± 0.23	139.4 ± 0.23	132.0 ± 0.20	128.8 ± 0.15	120.2 ± 0.2	0.42
K (mEq/L)	5.0 ± 0.05	13.2 ± 0.03	22.8 ± 0.04	22.4 ± 0.10	22.6 ± 0.07	<0.05
Cu (µg/dL)	81.0 ± 0.16	142.0 ± 0.16	154.0 ± 0.10	149.0 ± 0.13	167.0 ± 0.19	<0.05
Cr (µg/L)	2.2 ± 0.01	4.2 ± 0.05	4.9 ± 0.09	4.6 ± 0.07	5.8 ± 0.04	<0.05
Se (µg/L)	178.2 ± 0.31	77.6 ± 0.10	52.2 ± 0.25	56.4 ± 0.10	47.3 ± 0.20	<0.05
Pb (µg/L)	19.3 ± 0.1	40.2 ± 0.19	156.3 ± 0.17	161.2 ± 0.17	175.4 ± 0.2	<0.05

$p < 0.05$ value denotes significance between groups

Table 8: Semen parameters with trace metals concentration in seminal plasma of the study participants

Variables	Sperm count		Sperm motility		Sperm morphology	
	Pearson correlation	p value	Pearson correlation	p value	Pearson correlation	p value
Ca (mg/dL)	0.67	<0.01	0.79	<0.01	0.45	<0.01
Mg (mEq/L)	0.23	0.78	0.48	<0.01	0.61	<0.01
Na (mEq/L)	–0.19	0.13	–0.35	<0.01	–0.14	0.23
K (mEq/L)	–0.47	<0.01	–0.16	0.81	–0.15	0.56
Zn (mg/dL)	0.60	<0.01	0.71	<0.01	0.31	<0.05
Cu (μg/dL)	0.74	<0.01	0.35	0.55	0.12	0.89
Cr (μg/L)	–0.57	<0.01	–0.36	<0.01	–0.28	<0.05
Se (μg/L)	0.73	<0.01	0.65	<0.01	0.16	0.50
Pb (μg/L)	–0.71	<0.01	–0.20	0.19	–0.57	<0.01

Figure 15: Mean calcium, magnesium and zinc level in seminal plasma of the study participants among the different groups

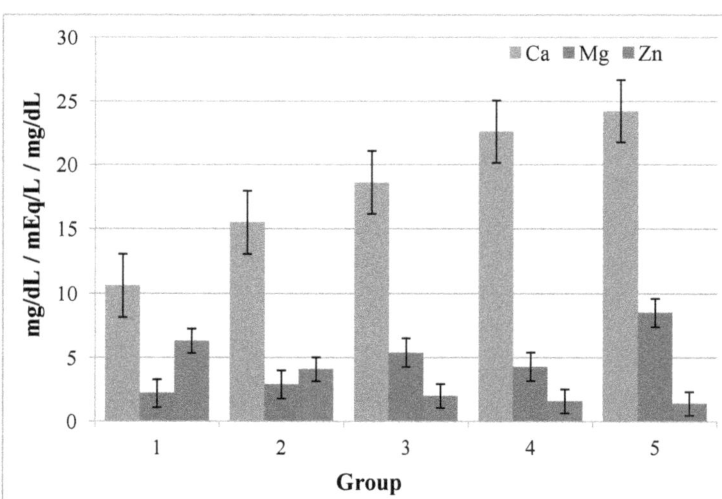

Figure 16: Scatter plots and linear regression lines of seminal plasma calcium level and semen parameters of the study participants

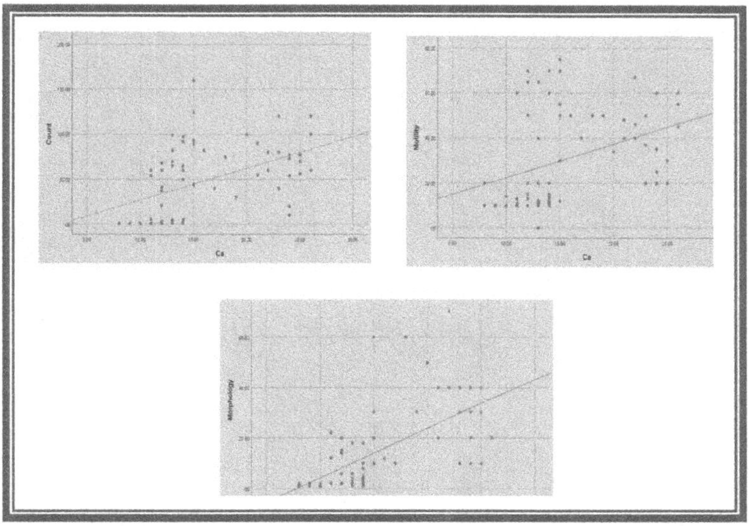

Figure 17: Scatter plots and linear regression lines of seminal plasma magnesium level and semen parameters of the study participants

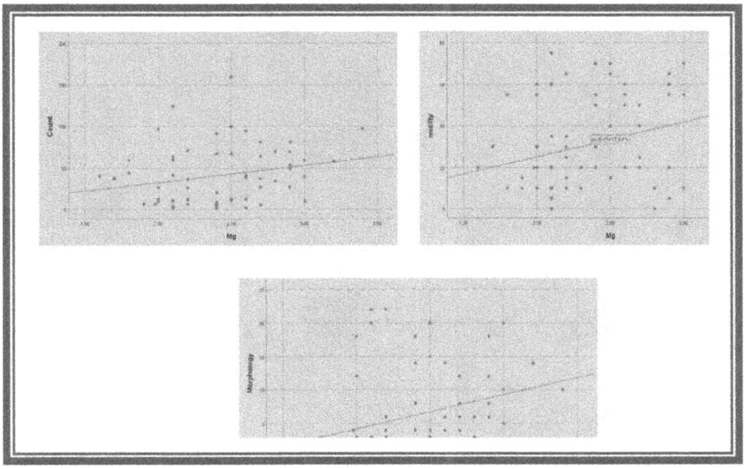

Figure 18: Scatter plots and linear regression lines of seminal plasma zinc level and semen parameters of the study participants

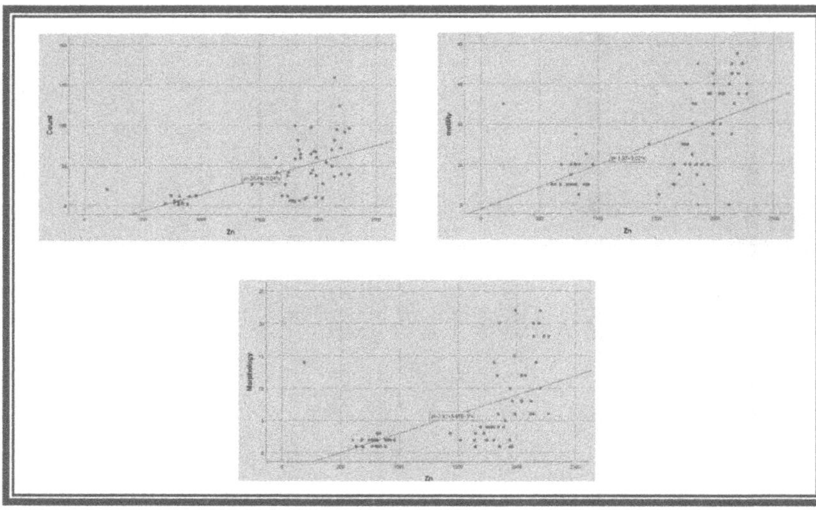

Figure 19: Mean sodium and potassium level in seminal plasma of the study participants among the different groups

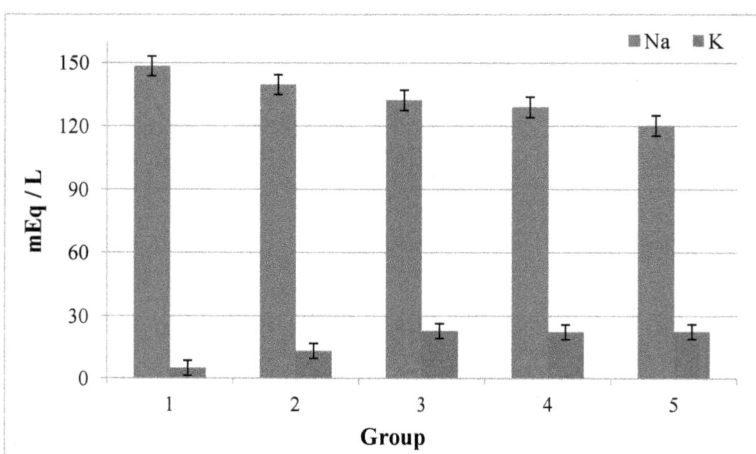

Figure 20: Scatter plots and linear regression lines of seminal plasma sodium level and semen parameters of the study participants

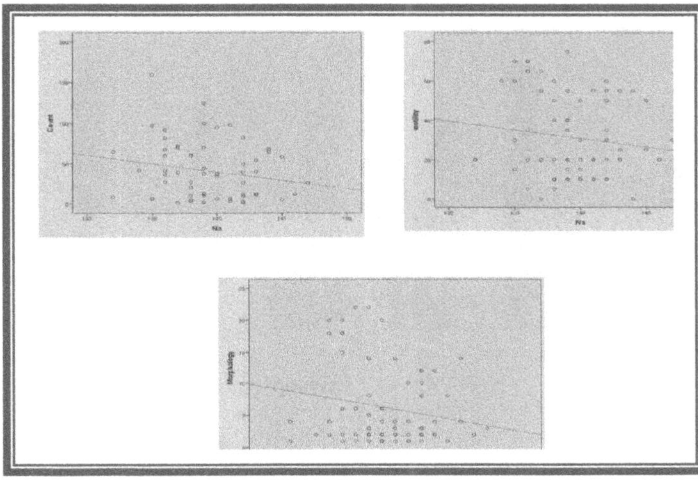

Figure 21: Scatter plots and linear regression lines of seminal plasma potassium level and semen parameters of the study participants

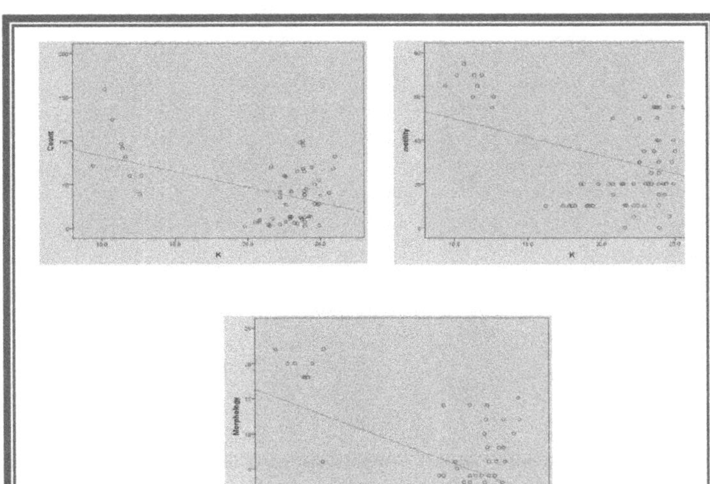

Figure 22: Mean copper and selenium level in seminal plasma of the study participants among the different groups

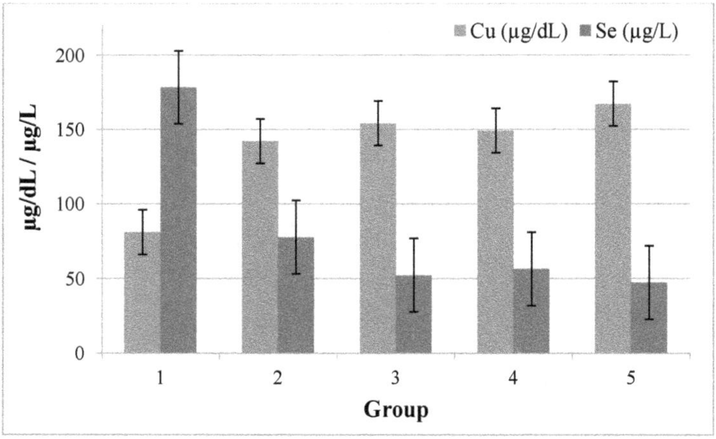

Figure 23: Scatter plots and linear regression lines of seminal plasma copper level and semen parameters of the study participants

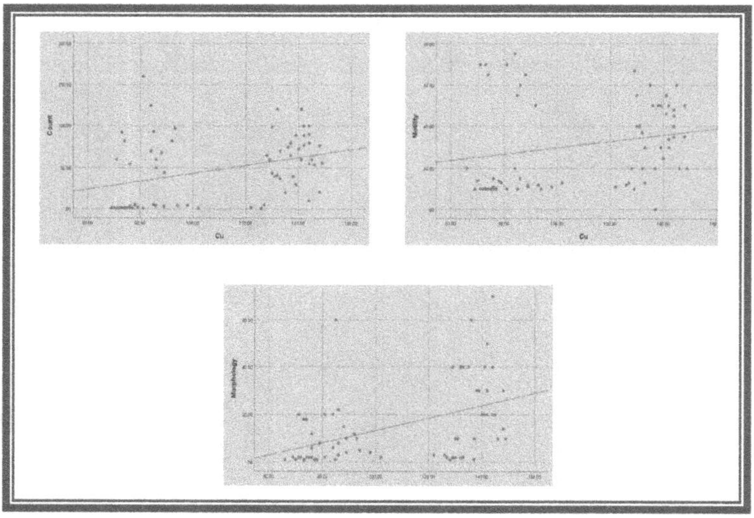

Figure 24: Scatter plots and linear regression lines of seminal plasma selenium level and semen parameters of the study participants

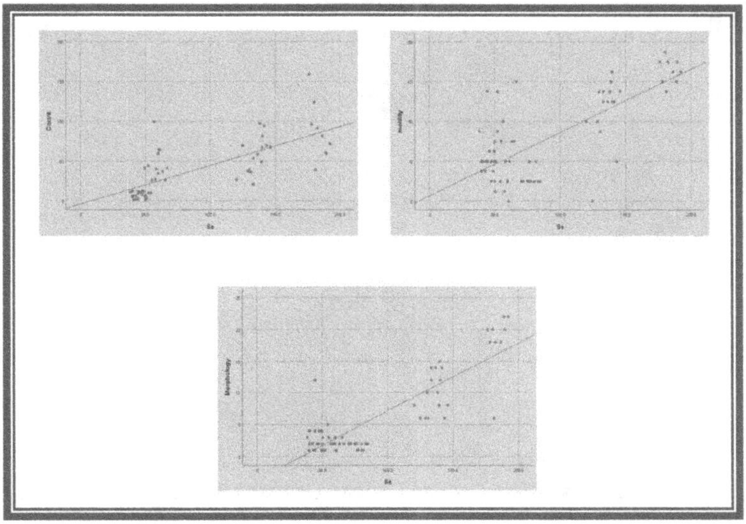

Figure 25: Mean chromium and lead level in seminal plasma of the study participants among the different groups

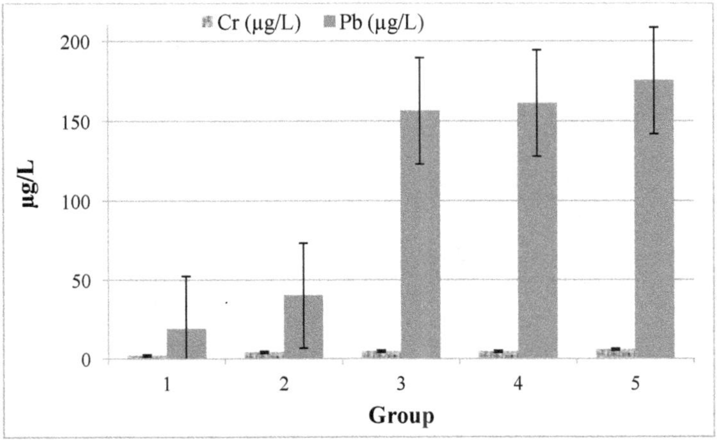

Figure 26: Scatter plots and linear regression lines of seminal plasma chromium level and semen parameters of the study participants

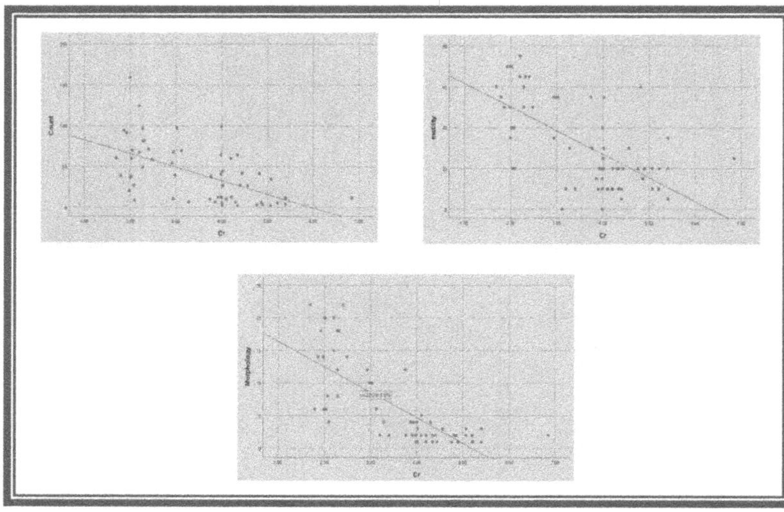

Figure 27: Scatter plots and linear regression lines of seminal plasma lead level and semen parameters of the study participants

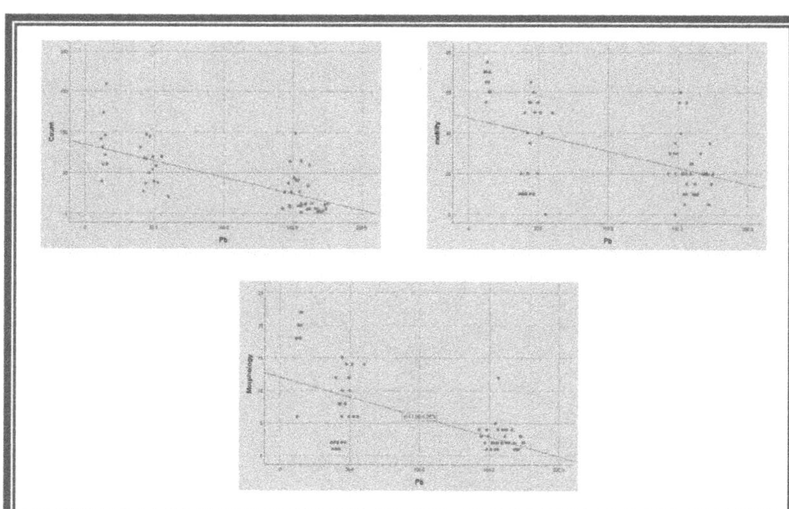

4.4 Hormones

4.4.1 Thyroid stimulating hormone (TSH)

Hormones play a major role in reproduction. Even it is trace in human body it plays a vital role in reproduction. The hormone profile of the participants was evaluated in blood serum. **Table 9** shows the hormone profile of participants and results shows that the mean TSH was 2.5 μIU/mL, 2.2 μIU/mL, 6.5 μIU/mL, 7.4 μIU/mL and 10.0 μIU/mL in groups 1–5, respectively (**Figure 28**).

Pearson correlation was applied to study the association between the TSH and semen parameters of the study groups (**Table 10**) and the results shows that mean sperm count ($r = -0.20$, $p<0.05$), sperm motility ($r = -0.99$, $p<0.05$) and sperm morphology ($r = -0.15$, $p<0.05$) shows a negative correlation with TSH level (**Figure 29**). It was clear from figure that TSH concentration was found elevated in group 3–5 compare to groups 1 & 2.

Similar finding was observed by Rajender *et al.*, (2011) and Sengupta (2013) to study impact of TSH on the male reproductive system was examined and results show that abnormal concentration of TSH lead to decreased sexual activity and poor semen quality, but Carani *et al.*, (2005) states that the sexual dysfunction is multi factorial, it is not necessary that all abnormal groups have hyper or hypothyroidism. Supportive study was conducted by Sharma *et al.*, (2012) found abnormal ranges of TSH were observed in poor semen quality participants compare to the normal group. Similar to our results found by Sarma *et al.*, (2017) observed negative correlation of TSH level with sperm count ($r = -0.73$, $p<0.05$).

Hyper or hypothyroidism is not very common in male, only 0.1% of the male in general population might have a thyroid problem (Krassas and Perros, 2003). Studies show that hypothyroidism (Krassas and Pontikides, 2004 & Hernandez *et al.*, 1990) and hyperthyroidism (Clyde *et al.*, 1976 and Rijntjes *et al.*, 2008) shows negative influence on semen parameters particularly count and motility. Study examines the relationship between spermatogenesis and hyperthyroidism in 21 patients and found that 43% of patients with low sperm counts and 61.9% of patients was with poor motility rate (Abalovich *et al.*, 1999).

4.4.2 Follicle stimulating hormone (FSH)

FSH plays an important role in induction and maintenance of spermatogenesis in male, the abnormal concentration of FSH leads to male infertility. From the **Table 9** it was evident that the mean FSH was 5.1 mIU/mL (Group1), 4.9 mIU/mL (Group 2), 12.1 mIU/mL (Group 3), 14.6 mIU/mL (Group 4) and 16.8 mIU/mL (Group 5) respectively. From the graphical presentation in **Figure 28** shows that the mean FSH was found significantly higher in group 2–5 compared to group 1. Scatter plots shows that mean sperm count ($r = -0.32$, $p<0.05$), sperm motility ($r = -0.12$, $p<0.05$), and sperm morphology ($r = -0.11$, $p<0.05$) shows a negative correlation with FSH level (**Figure 30**).

Elevated levels of FSH lead to a reduction in testosterone level results in testicular failure and lower level lead to hypogonadotropic hypogonadism (HH) and showed improvement in semen parameters after enhancing the FSH level (Rastrelli *et al.*, 2014). Uhler *et al.*, (2003) found no significant relationship between FSH level in pregnant and non-pregnant couple groups. In our study blood sample was collected at a single point at different timings based on participants visiting time. Carlsen *et al.*, (1999) have found elevated inhibin B level in the early morning and shown decline in concentration at afternoon and similar trend was also observed for FSH (Veldhuis *et al.*, 1987). A study conducted in 161 oligozoospermic men found normal level of LH and T, but FSH levels show a negative association with sperm count (Subhan *et al.*, 1995), which supports our findings. Another study observed 40% of higher FSH level in the infertile group compared to the normal group. Multiple regression models show that poor sperm morphology and motility were found with elevated FSH in the infertile group (Meeker *et al.*, 2007). Uhler *et al.*, (2003) conducted a study to examine the relationship with hormone profile and semen parameters in normal couples. Authors conclude that there was no significant difference in FSH between pregnant and non-pregnant group. A cross sectional study was conducted in infertile and fertile group. Participants were divided based on BMI as normal and overweight/obese. The result found that BMI shows a positive relationship with FSH and negative relationship with semen parameters from both infertile and fertile group (Khatoon *et al.*, 2014). Madhusoodanan *et al.*, (2020) conducted in men who underwent microscopic subinguinal varicocelectomy and results show a significant correlation between sperm counts and pre-operative FSH ($r = -0.31$, $p<0.05$). Supportive study was done by Corinne *et al.*, (2020) found a negative correlation between FSH and semen parameters in male partners of infertile couples.

4.4.3 Luteinizing hormone (LH)

The production of testosterone by leydig cells are initiated through LH, which plays an important role in sperm production. Higher and lower concentration of LH was directly affecting the semen parameters lead to male infertility (Ramanujam *et al.*, 2000). **Figure 31** shows that the mean LH level was 4.6 mIU/mL, 4.5 mIU/mL, 8.6 mIU/mL, 10.0 mIU/mL and 12.3 IU/mL in groups 1–5, respectively. **Figure 32** shows that the mean sperm count ($r = -0.26$, $p<0.05$), sperm motility ($r = -0.15$, $p<0.05$) and sperm morphology ($r = -0.11$, $p>0.05$), shows a negative correlation with LH level.

A study shows participants with Klinefelter's syndrome shows elevated LH levels lead to hypoandrogenism (Lanfranco *et al.*, 2004). Urry *et al.*, (1976) observed higher concentration of LH in the male with sperm counts of $<10 \times 10^6$/mL. Sheth *et al.*, (1976); Biswas *et al.*, (1978) found several fold higher concentration of LH in seminal plasma when compare to serum and also found the concentration was lower in azoospermia compared to oligozoospermia and normozoospermia group. Similar to our results the Bennet *et al.*, (1991) observed high LH level in oligozoospermia when compared to normozoospermia group. This shows that higher LH concentration leads to male infertility. Weiss *et al.*, (1992) identified molecular variants of LH and these variants shows associated with male infertility. Studies show that abnormal LH concentration was found in the seminal plasma of participants with varicocele (Abdalla *et al.*, 1981 and Stewart, 1974). A comparative cross-sectional study was conducted in 355 males of infertile couple's shows that 79.1% of males having abnormal LH level also found with abnormal semen parameters (Omo-Aghoja *et al.*, 2017). Hofny *et al.*, (2010) state that the higher BMI is one of the major risk factor for abnormal semen parameters. In this study found that obese oligozoospermia group shows abnormal LH level compared to normal group. This study shows a negative correlation of LH with sperm count ($r = -0.41$, $p<0.05$), motility ($r = -043$, $p<0.05$) and morphology ($r = -0.04$, $p<0.05$), which supports our findings. Ozdemir *et al.*, (2016) conducted a cross-sectional study in 198 infertile males shows that level of LH shows significant differences with semen parameters compared to control group. Jeng *et al.*, (2013) reported there is no significant difference in LH level among the smoker and non-smokers and also not found any association with semen parameters. Jorgensen *et al.*, (2016) conducted study in Denmark, Estonia, Finland, Germany, Latvia, Lithuania and Spain reported a negative correlation between LH and semen parameters.

4.4.4 Prolactin (PRL)

Exact role of prolactin in male reproduction health remains unclear. The mean PRL was 10.3 ng/mL in group 1, 12.2 ng/mL in group 2, 14.9 ng/mL in group 3, 20.4 ng/mL in group 4 and 25.4 ng/mL in group 5 (**Figure 31**). Data from the scatter plots shows that the mean sperm count ($r = -0.16$, $p<0.05$), sperm motility ($r = -0.09$, $p<0.05$) and sperm morphology ($r = -0.12$, $p>0.05$) shows a negative correlation with PRL level (**Figure 33**).

In men high level of prolactin called hyperprolactinaemia lead to decreasing in sex drive and erection (Biller *et al.*, 1999); but Lotti *et al.*, (2013) not found any significant correlation between prolactin and erectile function. The impact of hyperprolactinaemia on male reproductive health and infertile was examined by many studies (Micic *et al.*, 1985). Gonzales *et al.*, (1992) found higher prolactin levels in blood serum of azoospermia compare to normozoospermia similar findings was also observed in our study but studies conducted by Keskin *et al.*, (2015) showed that there was no correlation between prolactin levels and semen parameters between normal and abnormal group. Studies conducted by Polishuk *et al.*, (1975) observed significant improvement in semen parameter after suppression of prolactin by bromocriptine in oligozoospermia group. A comparative cross-sectional study conducted in 355 males of infertile couples shows that 86.0% of males having abnormal prolactin level also found with abnormal semen parameters ($p= 0.004$; or 3.50, CI-1.43-8.55), (Omo-Aghoja *et al.*, 2017). A study conducted in 1465 patients to find the association between hyperprolactinemia and semen parameters. Results show that 85 patients detected with hyperprolactinemia with abnormal semen parameters but the association was very weak (Alici *et al.*, 1998). Al-Daghistani *et al.*, (2006) conducted study in 120 patients to study the association between PRL and semen parameters. Patients were grouped into asthenozoospermia, oligozoospermia, severe oligozoospermia and azoospermia. Results show that the PRL level was found abnormal concentration in all study groups and shows a negative impact on semen parameters, which support our results. Ahmed N and Ahmed H, (2017) conducted a study with 212 males and divide them in hyperprolactinemia and normal prolactin group. Results show that there was significant negative correlation between prolactin and semen parameters, which support our findings.

4.4.5 Testosterone (TST)

Testosterone (TST) is an important male hormone play a vital role in reproductive health. Abnormal levels may affect the sex drive and semen quality. The mean TST level was 840.1 ng/dL in group 1, 629.9 ng/dL in group 2, 440.3 ng/dL in group 3, 412.5 ng/dL in group 4 and 338.8 ng/dL in group 5, respectively. **Figure 34** shows that TST level was higher in group 2-5, when compared with group 1. Pearson correlation was applied to examine the correlation between TST level and semen parameters, the results shows that the mean sperm count ($r= 0.47$, $p<0.05$), sperm motility ($r= 0.35$, $p<0.05$) and sperm morphology ($r= -0.25$, $p>0.05$), shows a positive correlation with TST level (**Figure 35**).

Testosterone is not only hormone involved in sperm production, it was simulated by other sex hormones. The level of TST may be higher in seminal plasma compared to serum. Studies show that normozoospermia converted to azoospermia by reduction of 65% of sperm count within 4 month use of testosterone treatment (WHO task force on male infertility, 1996). Study conducted by Babu *et al.*, (2004) observed significantly higher level of LH and FSH in infertile compare with fertile group, but there were no significant differences in TST level between the study groups. In contrast, study conducted by Ismael *et al.*, (2017) found a higher level of TST in fertile men compare to infertile men also found significant differences in sperm count, motility and morphology. Abnormal testosterone level was associated with abnormal semen parameters in 94.4% of the 18 subjects affected, showing more than 9 folds odds of been associated with abnormal semen parameters ($p= 0.009$; OR 9.16, CI 1.20 - 69.69) (Omo-Aghoja *et al.*, 2017).

The mean TST level in the abnormal group was not within allowed range; Arafa *et al.*, (2008) observed significant reduction in TST level in azoospermic and oligozoospermic compare to control group which supports our results. Animal studies conducted shows reduction in TST and LH level, count and motility after food restriction (Rehm *et al.*, 2008 and Sitzmann *et al.*, 2010). Similar results were also found in humans were the TST level was significantly decreased in abnormal compared to control group after caloric restriction but not found significant changes in spermatogenesis (Cangemi *et al.*, 2010). Studies observed decreased TST level and sperm count in obese men (Hakonsen *et al.*, 2011) and found significant improvement after weight loss.

Table 9: Concentration of hormones in the blood serum of the study participants

Hormone	Group 1 (n=9) (Mean ± SEM)	Group 2 (n=16) (Mean ± SEM)	Group 3 (n=13) (Mean ± SEM)	Group 4 (n=10) (Mean ± SEM)	Group 5 (n=12) (Mean ± SEM)	p* value
TSH (μIU/mL)	2.5 ± 0.9	2.2 ± 0.9	6.5 ± 1.5	7.4 ± 0.8	10.0 ± 1.2	<0.05
FSH (mIU/mL)	5.1 ± 2.3	4.9 ± 2.9	12.1 ± 3.9	14.6 ± 9.8	16.8 ± 1.4	<0.05
LH (mIU/mL)	4.6 ± 2.0	4.5 ± 1.5	8.6 ± 1.2	10.0 ± 2.8	12.3 ± 3.4	<0.05
PRL (ng/mL)	10.3 ± 3.8	12.2 ± 5.9	14.9 ± 6.6	20.4 ± 9.6	25.4 ± 4.6	<0.05
TST (ng/dL)	840.1 ± 68.4	629.9 ± 41.5	440.3 ± 26.3	412.5 ± 22.0	338.8 ± 62.2	<0.05

Table 10: Association of semen parameters with hormones concentration of the study participants

Variables	Sperm count		Sperm motility		Sperm morphology	
	Pearson correlation	p value	Pearson correlation	p value	Pearson correlation	p value
TSH (μIU/mL)	–0.20	<0.05	–0.99	<0.05	–0.15	<0.05
FSH (mIU/mL)	–0.32	<0.05	–0.12	<0.05	–0.11	<0.05
LH (mIU/mL)	–0.26	<0.05	–0.15	<0.05	–0.11	0.38
PRL (ng/mL)	–0.16	<0.05	–0.09	<0.05	–0.12	<0.05
TST (ng/dL)	0.47	<0.05	0.35	<0.05	0.25	<0.05

Figure 28: Mean TSH and FSH level in blood serum of the study participants among the different groups

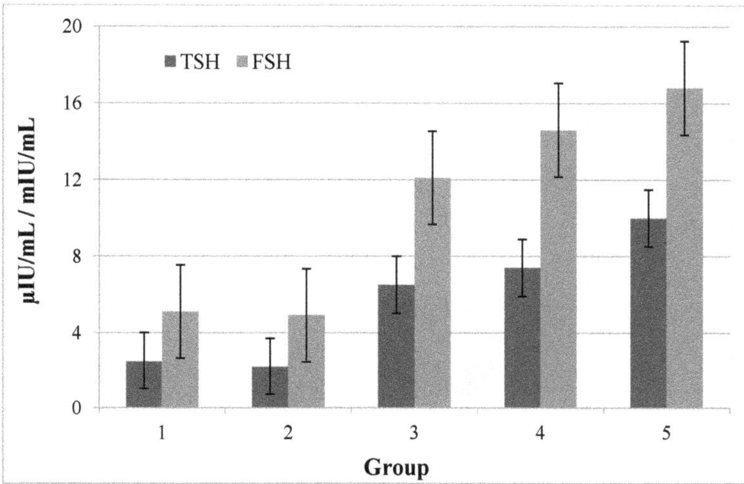

Figure 29: Scatter plots and linear regression lines of TSH level and semen parameters of the study participants

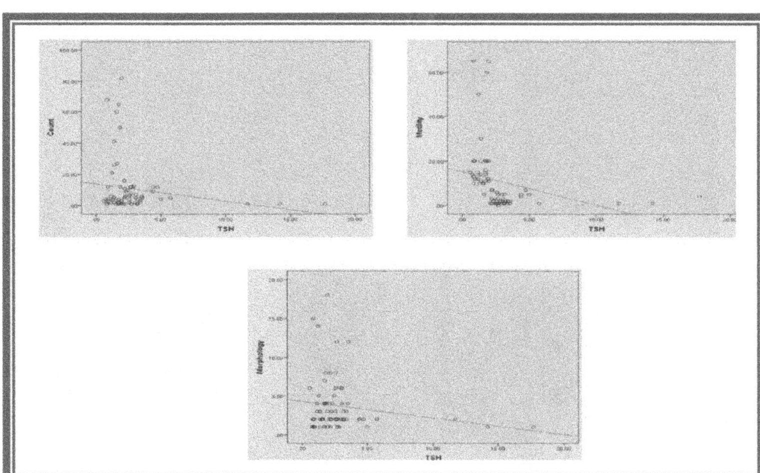

Figure 30: Scatter plots and linear regression lines of FSH level and semen parameters of the study participants

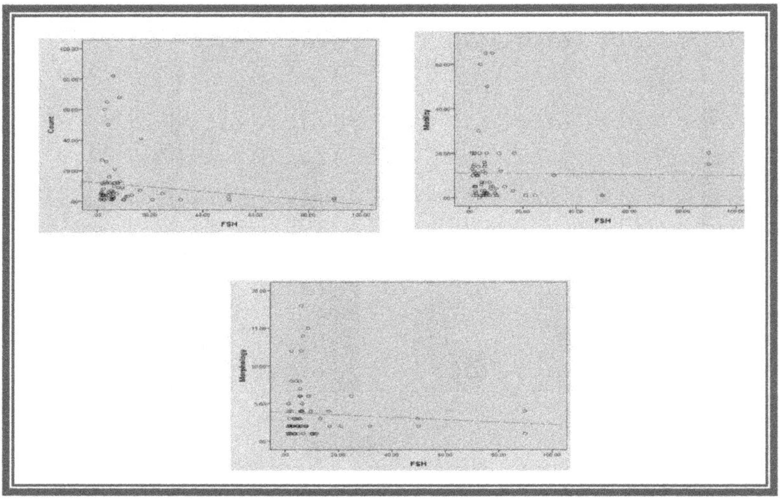

Figure 31: Mean LH and PRL level in blood serum of the study participants among the different groups

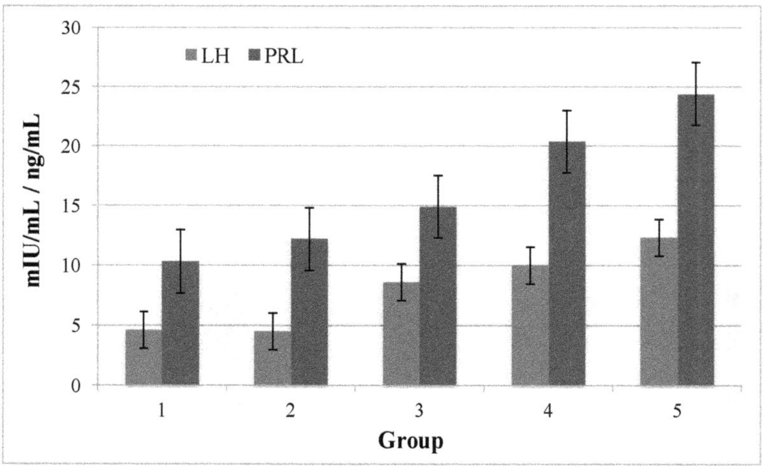

Figure 32: Scatter plots and linear regression lines of LH level and semen parameters of the study participants

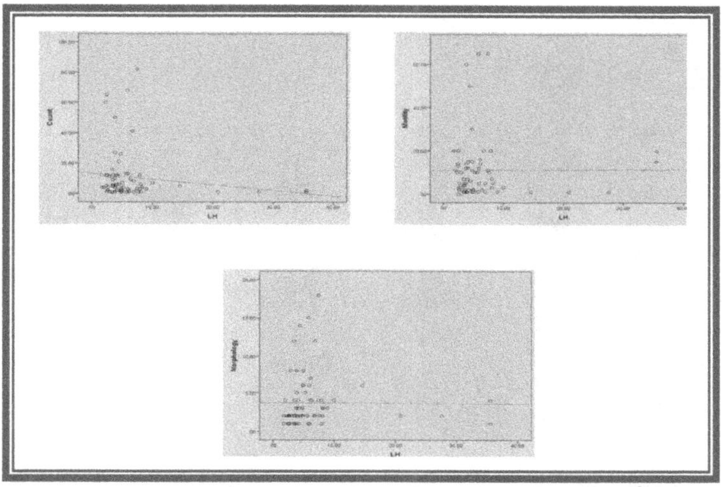

Figure 33: Scatter plots and linear regression lines of PRL level and semen parameters of the study participants

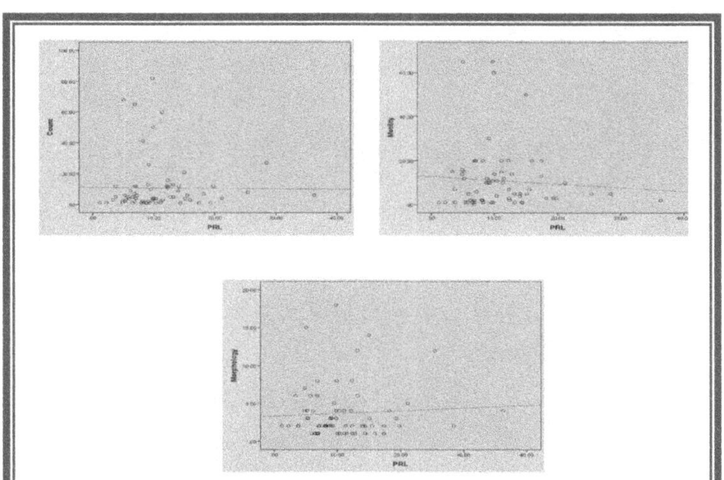

Figure 34: Mean TST level in blood serum of the study participants among the different groups

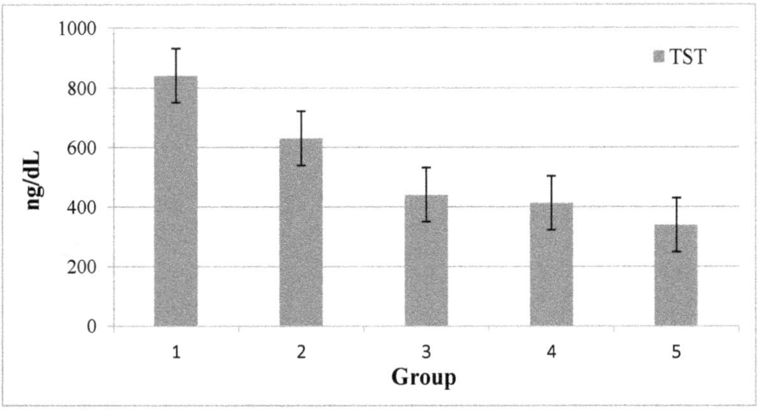

Figure 35: Scatter plots and linear regression lines of TST level and semen parameters of the study participants

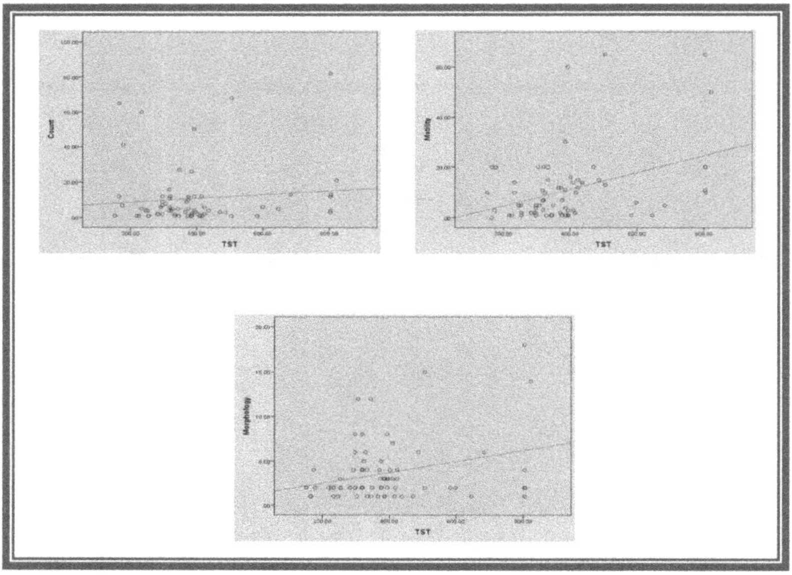

4.5.1 Association of occupation and semen quality

Association of semen parameters with behavior measures of the study participants indicated in **Table 11**. Based on the occupation, the participants were divided into 2 groups (IT and other workers). From **Table 12**, it was clear that the mean sperm count was higher in IT group (38.3 million/mL) and lower (36.6 million/mL) other industries group. Mean cell motility was observed as 30.2% and 28.9% in IT and other industries respectively. Higher normal morphology was found in IT (5.2%) and compared to other industries (5.0%) (**Figure 36**). The Pearson correlation was applied to examine the correlation of occupation and semen parameters and results show that mean sperm count ($r= -0.58$, $p<0.05$), sperm motility ($r= -0.09$, $p<0.05$) and Sperm morphology ($r= -0.16$, $p<0.05$) was showing negative effect with occupation of the study participants.

A study shows that 83.2% of workers were with abnormal sperm count with abnormal sperm motility when compared to control group, which supports our findings (Wadhwa *et al.*, 2019). Studies show that the worker in foundries, ceramic, bakers, welding industries was exposed high heat and stress lead to low sperm count and motility (Tas *et al.*, 1996 & Saradha and Mathur, 2006). Studies show that scrotal temperature of office clerks, drivers and computer operators was observed high and leads to abnormal semen parameters and found higher prevalence rate in male infertility among these workers (Swan *et al.*, 2000 and Sheiner *et al.*, 2003). Wang *et al.*, (2015) conducted study in formaldehyde industries employees. The result shows that the formaldehyde index was observed high and shows negative correlation with motility ($\beta=-0.19$, $p=0.01$) and semen parameters. Vaziri *et al.*, (2011) were no statistically significant differences in semen quality and occupational categories. The sperm count and motility and other semen parameters was lower in painters and construction workers compared to other occupations (Sadighi *et al.*, 2003). In our study around 5% of participants were welders and shows poor semen quality, supportive study was conducted by Hjollund *et al.*, (1998).

4.5.2 Association of infertility duration and semen quality

Based on the duration of infertility, the participants were divided into 2 groups (<5 years and >5 years). From the **Table 13**, it was evident that the mean sperm count was higher in <5 years group (43.6 million/mL) and lower (36.6 million/mL) in >5 years group. Mean motility was observed at 32.7% and 29.9% in <5 years and >5 years, respectively. Higher normal morphology was found in <5 years (6.2%) and compared to >5 years (6.0%)

(**Figure 37**). The Pearson correlation was applied to examine the correlation of occupation and semen parameters and results shows that mean sperm count ($r= -0.80$, $p<0.05$), sperm motility ($r= -0.81$, $p<0.05$) and sperm morphology ($r= -0.84$, $p<0.05$) was showing significant negative effect with infertility duration of the study participants.

Only limited data is available on the relationship and infertility duration. Aafjes *et al.*, (1978) shows the good semen quality and high success pregnancy rate was observed in men with <2years of duration compared to >2 years which support our findings. Others studies observed a significant decrease in live birth to increase in fertility duration (Templeton *et al.*, 1996 and Snick *et al.*, 1997). Supportive studies show the negative correlation between infertility duration and semen parameters (Zorba *et al.*, 2009 and Al-Ghazo *et al.*, 2011). A web based survey study conducted in 701 participants examines the knowledge about factors associated with male infertility. Results show that better knowledge score was found in participants with <2years duration of infertility compared to >2 years of infertility duration (Daumler *et al.*, 2016). Few other studies also studied about the infertility duration and the male reproductive health (Eisenberg *et al.*, 2013 and Chachamovich *et al.*, 2010). Supportive to our results shown Boeri *et al.*, (2018), were found a negative impact on semen parameters with an increase in infertility duration in 207 patients and conclude that longer duration associated with azoospermia in the study population.

4.5.3 Association of stress and semen quality

Based on the level of stress the participants were group into low and high stress and the results show that the mean sperm count (62.0 million/mL) was observed maximum in low stress group compared to high stress (31.9 million/mL) (**Table 14**). Similarly the mean sperm motility was 38.1% in low stress and 28.4% in the high stress group. The mean sperm morphology was found maximum (8.2%) in low stress compared to high stress (5.1%) group (**Figure 38**). The scatter plots show that the mean sperm count ($r= -0.20$, $p<0.05$), sperm motility ($r= -0.39$, $p<0.05$) and sperm morphology ($r= -0.23$, $p<0.05$) was negatively correlated with stress among the study groups.

Stress is commonly observed in the infertility patients. There are many stress factors include, testing, treatments, and low sex drive, occupational and social pressure (Anderson *et al.*, 2010). Studies found that high stress reduce the LH and TST level lead to low semen quality (Gollenberg *et al.*, 2010 and Corona *et al.*, 2016). Data from perceived stress scale from infertile males show higher stress score and show a negative correlation with overall semen quality. Author found that a decrease in sperm count (39%), motility (48%) but no changes was observed in volume and morphology (Spielberger *et al.*, 1970 & Ragni and Caccamo, 1992). Studies found a higher level of stress in men undergoing fertility treatment (Bhongade *et al.*, 2015 and Nordkap *et al.*, 2015). Support findings were done by (Janevic *et al.*, 2014), observed a negative correlation between stress and semen parameters include count, motility and morphology, but contrast to our finding a study was not found any association between stress and semen parameters. This study found low stress score with poor semen quality (Hjollund *et al.*, 2004). A stress on daily life in a family without exposure of stress environment may also shows a negative impact on semen parameters (Abu-Musa *et al.*, 2007) and other studies also found the association between stress and reproductive health (Eskiocak *et al.*, 2005 and Fukuda *et al.*, 1996). However, the research examining the association between psychosocial stress and semen quality has been inconsistent. A clinic based study examine the association between stressful life and semen quality and results show that only few life events like death in a family shows a negative correlation with sperm count, motility and morphology (Gollenberg *et al.*, 2010). A population based China study show that higher perceived stress score was associated with decreased sperm counts and morphology but not on motility (Li *et al.*, 2013).

4.5.4 Association of tight underwear and semen quality

Data on wearing tight underwear was collected from all participants (**Table 15**) and the results show that the mean sperm count (34.0 million/mL) was lower in tight underwear group compare to normal (41.5 million/mL). The mean sperm motility (30.7%) was observed higher in normal compared to tight underwear group (25.0%). Similarly, the mean morphology (3.6%) was lower in tight underwear group compared to normal (5.9%) (**Figure 39**). The Pearson correlation shows that the mean sperm count ($r= -0.13$, $p>0.05$), sperm motility ($r= -0.47$, $p>0.05$) and sperm morphology ($r= -0.16$, $p>0.05$) was non-significant weak negative correlation with wearing tight underwear among the study groups.

Several studies have been examines the relationship between loose/tight underwear and semen quality in infertile males (Oldereid *et al.*, 1991 and Pacey *et al.*, 2014). Studies have shown that the men wearing loose underwear shows better semen quality compare to tight underwear (Povey *et al.*, 2012 and Jurewicz *et al.*, 2014). Supportive study conducted by Sapra *et al.*, (2016) investigated the 501 male underwear type and wearing during day and night time on semen quality and the results found that only few changes was observed in semen parameters, but no significant differences with the control group. A similar finding was also observed by Oldereid *et al*., (1991); Munkelwitz and Gilbert, (1998) & Pacey *et al*., (2014). A few intervention studies conducted to examine the underwear association with semen quality. Underwear like device was wear by the fertile participants to hold the testis close to the body (Shafik, 1992 & Mieusset and Bujan, 1994). Some studies conducted by Shafik (1992); Mieusset and Bujan, (1994) & Ahmad *et al*., (2012) observed poor semen quality and higher scrotal temperature after using the device. Shafik (1992) reported infertile participants become azoospermia after several month of using device.

4.5.5 Association of smoking and semen quality

Table 16 shows that the low sperm count (36.5 million/mL), motility (26.8%), morphology (4.5%) was observed in smokers compared to non-smoker (count: 47.9 million/mL, motility: 38.5% and morphology: 8.6%). Pearson correlation shows that the sperm count ($r= -0.26$, $p<0.05$), sperm motility ($r= -0.16$, $p<0.05$) and sperm morphology ($r= -0.32$, $p<0.05$) was observed significant negative correlation with smoking among the study groups. It was observed that 11.1% (Group 1), 26.6% (Group 2), 24.4% (Group 3), 17.7% (Group 4) and 20.0% (Group 5) of smokers, respectively (**Figure 40**). It was observed that abnormal group 2–5 with highest percentage of smoker compared to normal group.

Studies showed that smoking directly influence the sperm motility and viability (Kulikauskas *et.al*., 1985 and Gaur *et al*., 2007). Smoking has been influence the sperm count in infertile group (Pasqualotto *et al*., 2006), also observed reduction in sperm count in healthy young smoker group (Richthoff *et al*., 2008). Chia *et al*., (1994) also reported similar results in 618 Chinese smoker males have lower sperm count, motility and morphology. Dose dependent study conducted in 358 Mexican males group based on the number of cigarettes smoked/day. The results show a negative correlation between smoking and semen parameters. The authors conclude that even a light smoker (<10 cigarettes/day) also shows significant differences in semen parameters (Merino *et al*., 1998). But some studies not found significant difference between smoking and semen parameters (Povey *et* al., 2012 and Hassa, *et al*., 2006). A study conducted in 166 couples ART observed low success rate in IVF, ICSI and live birth rate in male partner with smoking habit compared to non-smoking male partners (Fuentes *et al*., 2010). Few other studies also examine the effect of smoking on ART (Joesbury *et al*., 1998 and Zitzmann *et al*., 2003). Meta-analysis study was conducted by Li *et al*., (2011) analyzed 57 observational studies on smoking and semen parameters in both fertile and infertile male. Results show that smoking showing adverse effect on all sperm parameters. Kunzle *et al.*, (2003) reported the decrease in sperm count (17.5%), motility (16.6%) and density (15.3%) in infertile smokers compared to non-smoker.

4.5.6 Association of alcohol consumption and semen quality

Table 17 shows that the low sperm count (36.1 million/mL), motility (28.5%), morphology (5.3%) was observed in alcoholic compared to non-alcoholic participants (count: 55.8 million/mL, motility: 40.9% and morphology: 8.8%). Pearson correlation shows that the sperm count ($r = -0.24$, $p<0.05$), and sperm motility ($r = -0.31$, $p<0.05$) and sperm morphology ($r = -0.20$, $p<0.05$) was observed significant negative correlation with alcohol consumption among the study groups. It is evident from **Figure 41**, that among the study participants 11.2% in group 1, 22.5% in group 2, 17.5% in group 3, 20.0% in group 4 and 13.5% in group 5 was alcoholic.

Alcohol consumption shows negative impact at various levels in sperm production (Emanuele and Emanuele, 1998). A study conducted by Kuller *et al.*, (1978) observed very less spermatogenesis in men consumed more than 32 drinks per week and author also found reduction in spermatogenesis on daily drinkers. High consumption of alcohol shows direct impact of semen parameters (Jensen *et al.*, 2014 and Villalta *et al.*, 1997) but contrast results was observed by Li *et al.*, (2009). Study conducted in mice shows that absence of alcohol consumption showed improvement in spermatogenesis (Anderson *et al.*, 1985) and similar results also found in humans study observed significant improvement in semen parameters of azoospermia after stop consuming alcohol (Sermondade *et al.*, 2010).

Amount of alcohol intake per day negative correlates with all the three semen parameters in all groups, similar finding was observed by Gaur *et al.*, (2010) in asthenozoospermia, teratozoospermia and oligozoospermia. Six years follow up study conducted in chronic alcohol consumption males show a negative correlation with semen parameters. Author concludes that the participants was teratozoospermia at baseline and gradually changed as azoospermia. Improvement of semen was observed after withdrawal of alcohol consumption (Sermondad *et al.*, 2010). Similar to our findings, Studies conducted by Martini *et al.*, (2004) & Muthusami and Chinnaswamy (2005) shows a negative correlation between alcohol consumption and semen parameters, but contrast to our findings, studies conducted by Hansen *et al.*, (2012) and Teijon *et al.*, (2007) not found any association. Meta-analysis report of 15 cross sectional studies included nearly 16395 men shows that alcohol intake was directly affected by the semen volume (0.25 mL, 95% CI, 0.07 to 0.42) and normal morphology (1.87%, 95% CI, 0.86 to 2.88%) (Ricci *et al.*, 2017).

4.5.7 Association of food habit and semen quality

Table 18 shows that the low sperm count (43.7 million/mL), motility (36.9%) and morphology (7.0%), was observed in non-vegetarians compared to vegetarians (count: 44.1 million/mL, motility: 39.1% and morphology: 7.5%) (**Figure 42**). Pearson correlation shows that the sperm count ($r = 0.44$, $p < 0.05$), sperm motility ($r = 0.41$, $p < 0.05$) and sperm morphology ($r = 0.39$, $p < 0.05$) was observed significant correlation with food habit among the study groups.

Analysing the dietary patterns is very important parameter to describe the exact role of each nutrient in reproductive health. Few observational and invention studies examine the role of single nutrients on semen quality (Mendiola *et al.*, 2010 and Schowell *et al.*, 2014) few other used food products (Eslamian *et al.*, 2012; Eslamian *et al.*, 2016 and Mendiola *et al.*, 2009). Studies on investing the role of food habit and semen quality shows that few food shows protective effect on semen quality and few show reduced its quality (Salas-Huetos *et al.*, 2017). These contrast observational results may due that different studies conducted in various populations on different food habits. Study conducted by Eslamian *et al.*, (2016) found that western food habits was positive associated with asthenozoospermia and shows reduction in sperm concentration and morphology (Liu *et al.*, 2015), but Gaskins *et al.*, (2012) and Oostingh *et al.*, (2017) did not find such association between western diet and semen quality. Study reported that consumption of animal products like dairy, meat and red meat shows decline in semen quality (Salas-Huetos *et al.*, 2017). Studies shows that intake of low fat dairy products enhanced the semen quality, but shows decline with full fat dairy products (Afeiche *et al.*, 2013). Few studies also state that high intake of dairy products leads to oligoasthenoteratozoospermia and asthenozoospermia in men from infertile couples (Eslamian *et al.*, 2012 and Mendiola *et al.*, 2009). Animal products contains is lipophilic and accumulate high fat in the body affects the semen quality (Rozati *et al.*, 2002). Liu *et al.*, (2015) and Eslamian *et al.*, (2012) reported that sweet, snacks, sweetened drinks and carbohydrate food were associated with increase prevalence rate of male infertility. Liu *et al.*, (2015) show that there is no significant difference in semen parameter with vegetable and fruits consumption.

Table 11: Association of semen parameters with behavior measures of the study participants

Variables	Sperm count		Sperm motility		Sperm morphology	
	Pearson correlation	p value	Pearson correlation	p value	Pearson correlation	p value
Occupation	–0.58	0.05	–0.09	0.05	–0.16	0.05
Infertility duration	–0.80	0.51	-0.81	0.47	–0.84	0.94
Stress	–0.20	0.05	–0.39	0.05	–0.23	0.05
Tight underwear	–0.13	0.25	–0.47	0.72	–0.16	0.11
Smoking	–0.26	0.05	–0.16	0.22	–0.32	0.05
Alcohol	–0.24	0.05	–0.31	0.05	–0.20	0.05
Food habit	0.44	0.05	0.41	0.05	0.39	0.05

Table 12: Association of occupation semen parameters of the study participants

Semen parameters	IT (n = 31)	Other industries (n = 29)	p value
Count (million/mL)	38.3 ± 5.7	36.6 ± 6.2	<0.05
Motility (%)	30.2 ± 3.23	28.9 ± 5.01	<0.05
Morphology (%)	5.21 ± 0.89	5.05 ± 0.52	<0.05

Figure 36: Role of occupation in semen parameters of the study participants among the different groups.

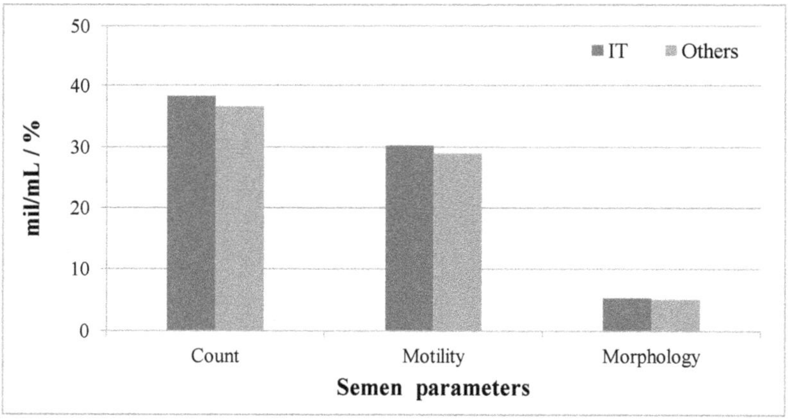

Table 13: Effect of infertility duration on semen parameters of the study participants

Semen parameters	<5 years (n = 40)	>5 years (n = 20)	p value
Count (million/mL)	43.6±5.3	36.6±8.7	<0.05
Motility (%)	32.7±3.3	29.9±3.88	<0.05
Morphology (%)	6.27±0.96	6.07±1.20	<0.05

Figure 37: Effect of infertility duration in semen parameters of the study participants among the different groups.

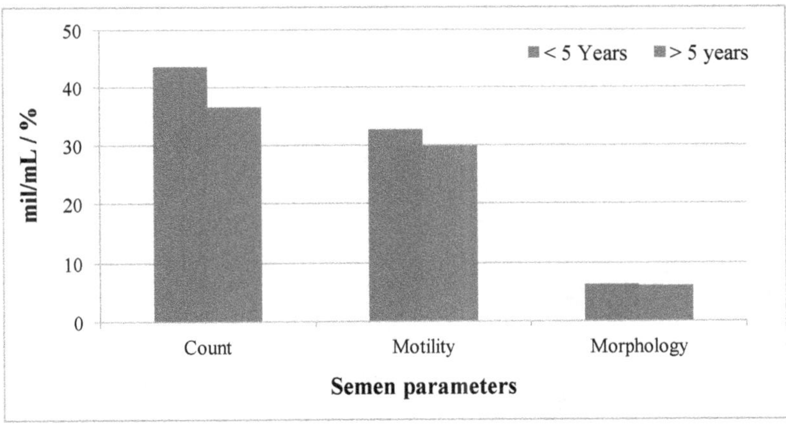

Table 14: Effect of stress on semen parameters of the study participants

Semen parameters	Low stress (n = 38)	High stress (n = 22)	p value
Count (million/mL)	62.0 ± 10.0	31.9 ± 4.29	<0.05
Motility (%)	38.1 ± 5.39	28.4 ± 2.73	<0.05
Morphology (%)	8.29 ± 1.64	5.19 ± 0.77	<0.05

Figure 38: Effect of stress on semen parameters of the study participants among the different groups.

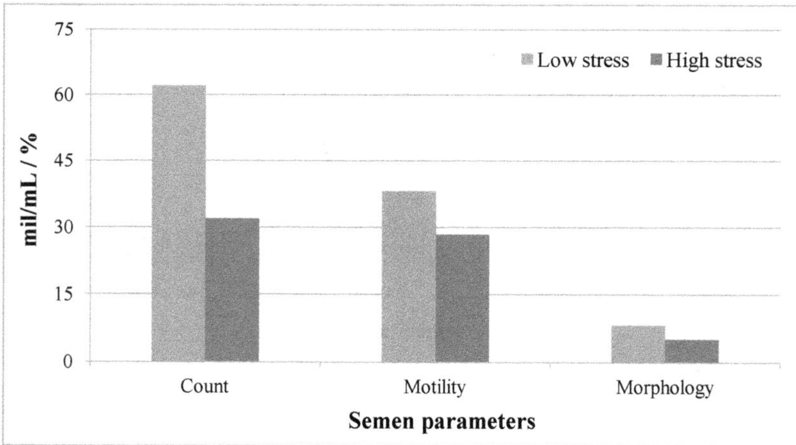

Table 15: Effect of tight underwear on semen parameters of the study participants

Semen parameters	No (n = 25)	Yes (n = 35)	p value
Count (million/mL)	41.5 ± 4.78	34.0 ± 10.9	<0.05
Motility (%)	30.7 ± 2.59	25.0 ± 12.5	<0.05
Morphology (%)	5.91 ± 0.73	3.62 ± 0.81	<0.05

Figure 39: Effect of tight underwear on semen parameters of the study participants among the different groups.

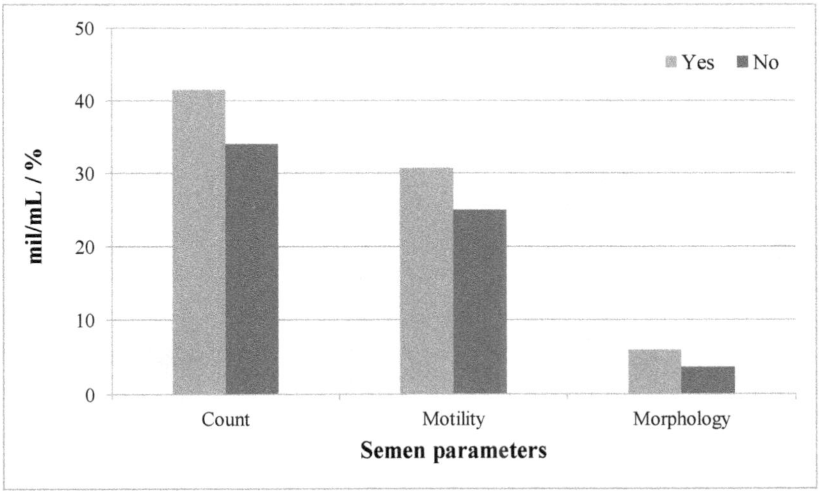

Table 16: Effect of smoking on semen parameters of the study participants

Semen parameters	Non-smoking (n = 15)	Smoking (n = 45)	p value
Count (million/mL)	47.9 ± 8.8	36.5 ± 4.7	<0.05
Motility (%)	38.5 ± 4.5	26.8 ± 2.80	<0.05
Morphology (%)	8.69 ± 1.52	4.58 ± 0.68	<0.05

Figure 40: Effect of smoking on semen parameters of the study participants among the different groups.

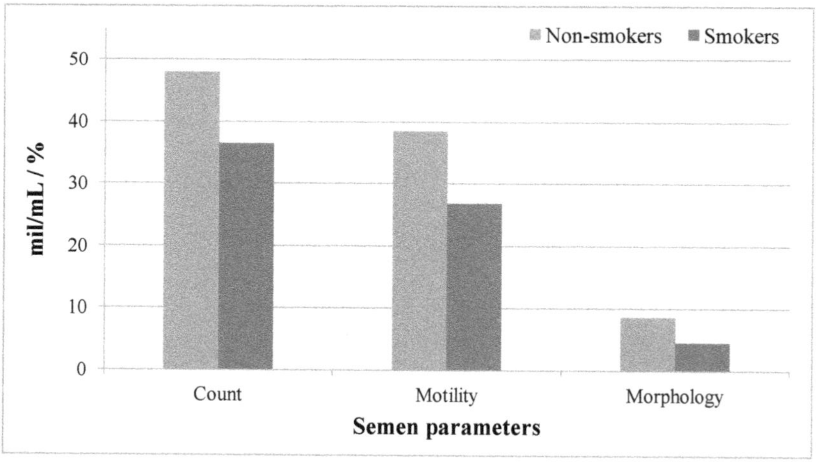

Table 17: Effect of alcohol consumption on semen parameters of the study participants

Semen parameters	Non-alcoholic (n = 20)	Alcoholic (n = 40)	p value
Count (million/mL)	55.8 ± 10.1	36.1 ± 4.98	<0.05
Motility (%)	40.9 ± 5.8	28.5 ± 2.71	<0.05
Morphology (%)	8.88 ± 1.9	5.30 ± 0.74	<0.05

Figure 41: Effect of alcohol consumption on semen parameters of the study participants among the different groups.

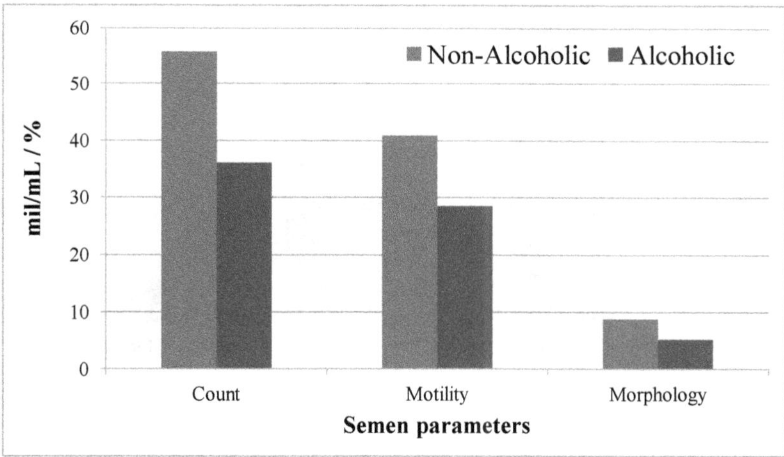

Table 18: Effect of food habit on semen parameters of the study participants

Semen parameters	Vegetarian (n=13)	Non-vegetarian (n=47)	p value
Count (million/mL)	44.1 ± 8.5	43.7 ± 3.36	<0.05
Motility (%)	39.1 ± 4.6	36.9 ± 7.01	<0.05
Morphology (%)	7.50 ± 2.2	7.00 ± 0.11	<0.05

Figure 42: Effect of food habit on semen parameters of the study participants among the different groups

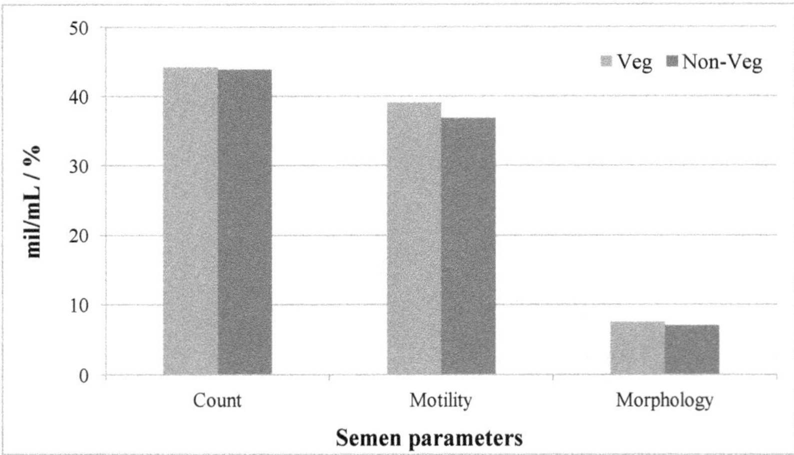

4.6 Association of vitamin D and semen parameters

The concentration of vitamin D of the participants in among the various groups was given in **Table 19**. It was found that the vitamin D concentration in semen plasma was observed as 72.1 ng/mL, 23.8 ng/mL, 20.4 ng/mL, 13.3 ng/mL and 18.0 ng/mL in groups 1–5, respectively (**Figure 43**). There is a significant difference in vitamin D concentration among groups 1–5. **Table 20** & **Figure 44** shows that mean sperm count ($r = 0.19$, $p<0.05$), sperm motility ($r = 0.09$, $p>0.05$); and morphology ($r = 0.19$, $p<0.05$) shows significant positive correlation with vitamin D level.

Studies conducted in animals and humans reported that vitamin D is necessary for male reproduction (Jensen *et al.*, 2010 and Mahmoudi *et al.*, 2013). Below 10 ng/mL is considered as vitamin D deficiency; 11–31 ng/mL is insufficiency, 31 to 100 ng/mL is generally accepted as sufficient and above 100 ng/mL is considered as toxicity (Holick *et al.*, 2011). In this study we observed our participants from group 2–5 were with insufficient vitamin D. Recent studies have observed the correlation between semen quality and vitamin D (Aquila *et al.*, 2009; Jensen, 2014 and Boisen *et al.*, 2016).

Uhland *et al.*, (1992) reported the effect the fertility was improved in rats vitamin D deficient rats after the treatment with vitamin D. Study shows a positive correlation with vitamin D deficiency and lower sperm count, morphology (Jensen *et al.*, 2011) which is support to our findings that all abnormal group participants shows a lower vitamin D level. Hammoud *et al.*, (2012) illustrated in that vitamin D lower than 20 ng/mL and above 50 ng/mL show significant changes in semen parameters. Similar observation was found in group 4 and 5 participants. Supportive study done by Alzoubi *et al.*, (2017) found a positive relationship in the sperm count ($r = 0.2428$, $p = 0.0084$), motility ($r = 0.2827$, $p = 0.0020$) and morphology ($r = 0.3554$, $p = < 0.0001$). Pre-clinical (Sood *et al.*, 1995; Hirai *et al.*, 2009 and Kwiecinksi *et al.*, 1989), clinical (Foresta *et al.*, 2011) and *in vitro* (Nangia *et al.*, 2007) studies shows a correlation between vitamin D and semen parameters. Studies show that positive correlation with sperm count (Jensen *et al.*, 2016 and Rehman *et al.*, 2018) motility (Deng *et al.*, 2014 and Abbasihormozi *et al.*, 2017) and morphology (Rehman *et al.*, 2018 and Akhavizadegan *et al.*, 2017).

Table 19: Concentration of vitamin D of the study participants among the study groups

Group	Vitamin D (Mean ± SEM)	p value
1	72.1 ± 3.5	<0.05
2	23.8 ± 2.5	
3	20.4 ± 13.7	
4	13.3 ± 1.2	
5	18.0 ± 7.3	

Table 20: Correlation of vitamin D and semen parameters of the study participants among the study groups

Parameters	Pearson correlation	p value
Sperm count	0.19	<0.05
Sperm motility	0.09	0.44
Sperm morphology	0.19	<0.05

Figure 43: Level of vitamin D of the study participants among the different groups

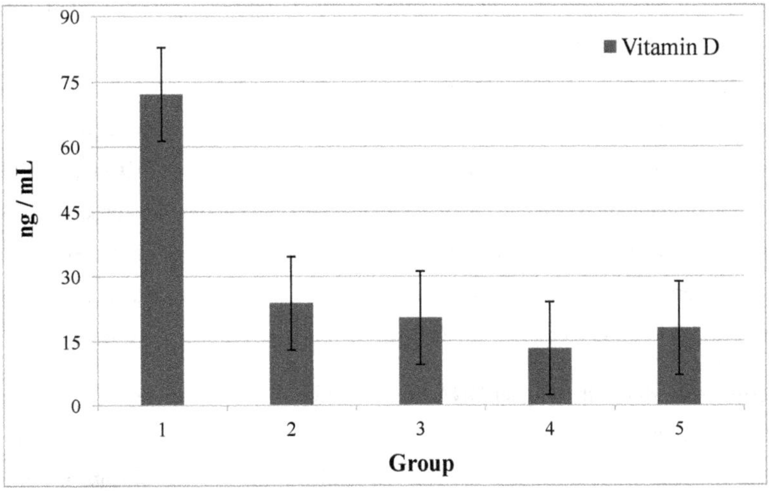

Figure 44: Scatter plots and linear regression lines of vitamin D and semen parameters

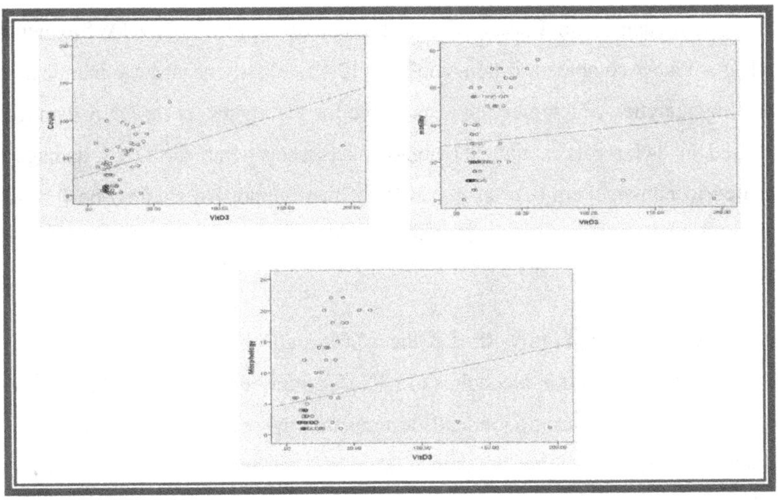

4.7 DNA fragmentation

The results of DNA fragmentation of the study participants with respect to age, BMI, smoking, alcohol consumption and stress were shown in **Table 21**. Microscopic images of DNA fragmentation was shown in **Plate 3**. It was observed that DNA fragmentation was found high (15.2%) in the older age group (41–50 years) compares to younger age group (20–30 years) (**Figure 45**). A similar result was found by Pino *et al.*, (2020) reported that the sperm DNA fragmentation was increased along with age. The author was observed 4.5 times more DNA fragmentation in men above 50 years compare to younger males. Similar studies were also observed by same findings which supports our results (Varshini *et al.*, 2012; Oliveira *et al.*, 2014 and Petersen *et al.*, 2018).

Figure 46 shows that higher DNA fragmentation was observed high (15.5%) in obese or overweight compare to normal BMI (11.6%) participants. Dupont *et al.,* (2013) reported that 2.5 times more DNA damage was observed in obese infertile participants. Other similar supportive findings show that the BMI shows a positive correlation with DNA fragmentation (Chavarro *et al.*, 2010; Hammiche *et al.*, 2011; Kort *et al.*, 2006; Tunc *et al.*, 2011; Rybar *et al.*, 2011; Fariello *et al.*, 2012 and La Vignera *et al.*, 2012).

It is evident from **Figure 47** that the maximum (15.2%) DNA fragmentation was found in smokers compared to non-smokers (12.6%). Many hazardous chemical substances present in cigarettes which may the responsible for the higher sperm DNA damage. A study conducted in 841 smokers and 287 non-smokers shows that the DNA damage was high compared to non-smokers (Cui *et al.*, 2016). Other supportive studies show similar results between smoker and non-smokers (Sepaniak *et al.*, 2004; Silver *et al.*, 2005 and Ozkosem *et al.*, 2015).

It is clear from **Figure 48** that the 15.0% of DNA fragmentation was observed in alcoholics compared to non-alcoholics (13.4%). A study conducted by Talebi *et al.*, (2011) reported that alcohol consumption leads to reduction in spermatogenesis and increased DNA fragmentation. Similar supportive studies show that alcohol consumption shows a positive correlation. A study shows that 49.6% of sperm DNA abnormalities index in drinkers compared to non-drinkers (33.9%) (Wiseman *et al.*, 1996). Few other studies show that DNA fragmentation associated with alcohol consumption (Anifandis *et al.*, 2014; Muratori *et al.*, 2016; Abarikwu *et al.*, 2016 and Hansen *et al.*, 2012).

Table 21: Association between DNA fragmentation and metabolic & behaviour parameters of the study participants

Variables	DNA fragmentation	p value
Age		
20–30 (n=21)	13.0 ± 1.5	<0.05
31–40 (n=30)	13.8 ± 0.24	
41–50 (n=09)	15.2 ± 0.55	
BMI		
<25 (n=27)	11.6 ± 1.8	<0.05
>25 (n=33)	14.5 ± 1.4	
Smoking		
Smoker (n=46)	15.2 ± 1.36	<0.05
Non-smoker (n=15)	12.6 ± 1.96	
Alcohol		
Alcoholic (n=40)	15.0 ± 1.19	<0.05
Non-alcoholic (n=20)	13.4 ± 2.79	

Figure 45: Association of age and DNA fragmentation of the study participants

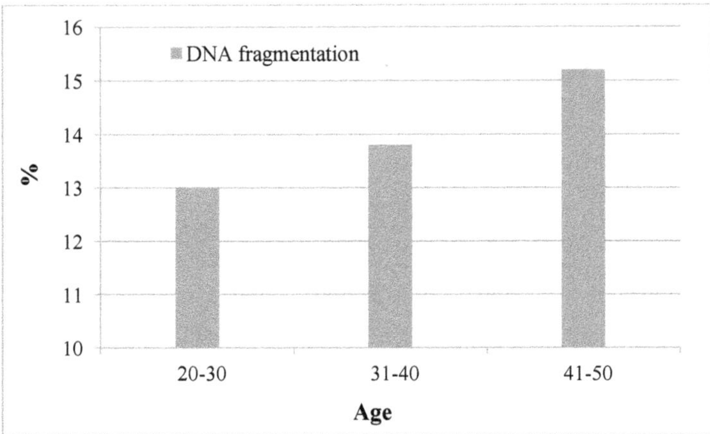

Figure 46: Association of BMI and DNA fragmentation of the study participants

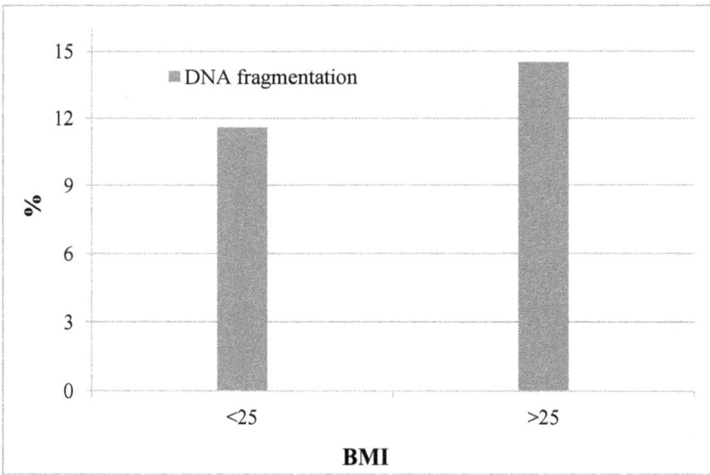

Figure 47: Association of smoking and DNA fragmentation of the study participants

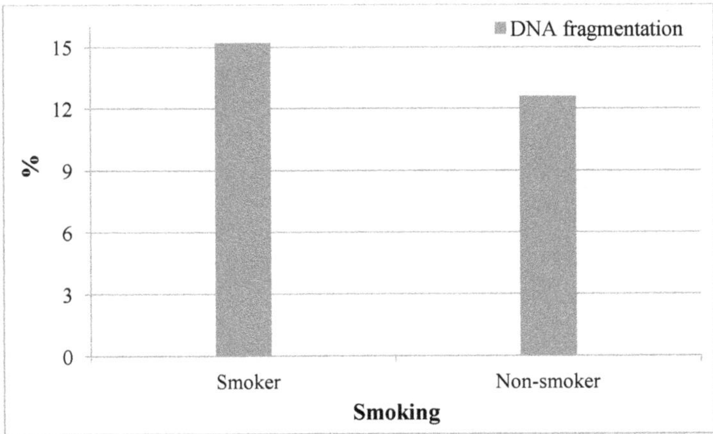

Figure 48: Association of alcohol consumption and DNA fragmentation of the study participants

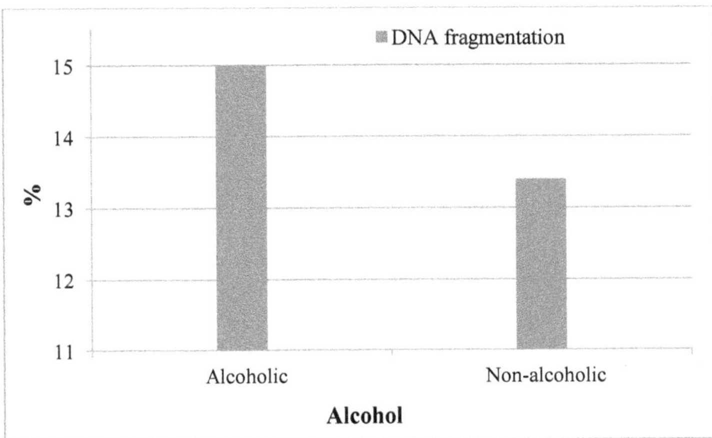

Plate 3: DNA fragmentation among the different study groups

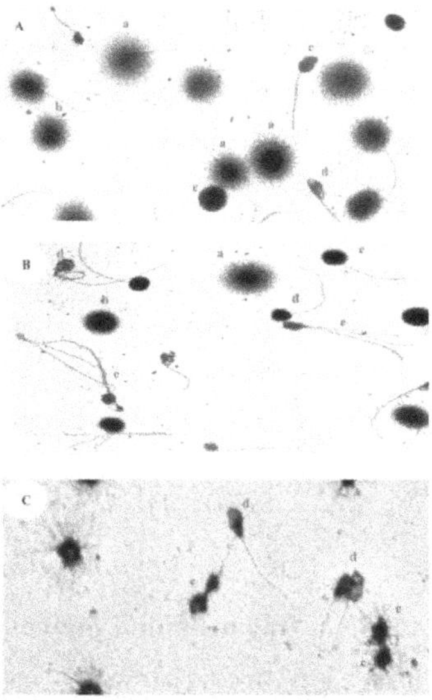

A. Normozoospermia B. Asthenozoospermia C. Asthenoteratozoospermia.
a. Big halo, b. Medium halo, c. Small halo, d. Without halo, e. Degraded

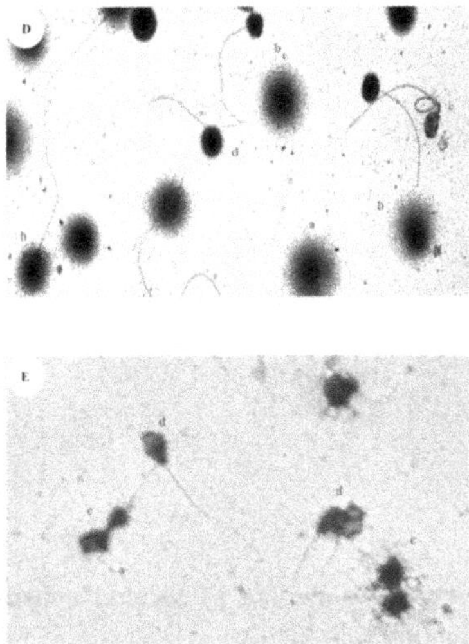

D. Oligoasthenozoospermia, E. Oligoasthenoteratozoospermia.
a. Big halo, b. Medium halo, c. Small halo, d. Without halo, e. Degraded

5.0 SUMMARY

- The present study was performed to analyze the role of trace metals on male infertility. Sixty infertile subjects were recruited from Kanmani Fertility Center Pvt. Ltd., Chennai, Tamilnadu, India. Participants were grouped based on sperm count, motility and morphology as per WHO criteria.

- The result demonstrates that among the study participants, 15.0% of them were normozoospermia, asthenozoospermia (26.6%), asthenoteratozoospermia (21.6%), oligoasthenozoospermia (16.6%), oligoasthenoteratozoospermia (20.0) respectively.

- Consequences of semen analysis include liquefaction, pH, sperm count, motility and morphology shows that participants from groups 2 to 5 show abnormal semen parameters when compared to the normal group 1.

- The mean liquefaction time was 28.5 minutes, 28.1 minutes, 28.3 minutes, 27.3 minutes, and 24.8 minutes for groups 1–5, respectively, and the mean pH of the collected semen was 7.9, 7.8, 7.6, 7.8 and 7.2 in all 5 groups, respectively.

- The mean volume of semen was 4.1 mL, 3.2 mL, 3.0 mL, 3.7 mL, and 2.8 mL for the groups 1–5, respectively. The mean sperm count was 87.1 million/mL (group 1), 54.4 million/mL (group 2), 46.7 million/mL (group 3), 8.8 million/mL (group 4) and 6.3 million/mL (group 5) respectively.

- The motility of sperm was analyzed in all study participants and the results show that group 1 participants with 61.6%, followed by group 2 (41.2%), group 3 (22.3%), group 4 (24.5%) and group 5 (6.6%) of motile sperms respectively. The percentage of normal sperm morphology was recorded in all study participants. It was found that only 18.2%, 9.3%, 1.9%, 4.5% and 1.8% of normal sperms was found in groups 1–5, respectively.

- Association and correlation of anthropometric parameters with semen quality shows that age, body weight, BMI and blood pressure shows the negative correlation. The mean age of the study participant was 33.0 years, 37.1 years, 37.0 years, 34.3 years and 35.5 years from groups 1–5, respectively.

- The mean body weight of study participants was 73.6 Kg, 84.8 Kg, 95.7 Kg, 93.6 Kg, and 84.6 Kg from groups 1–5, respectively, and the mean BMI of the study participants was 23.2 Kg/m^2, 27.7 Kg/m^2, 30.8 Kg/m^2, 28.6 Kg/m^2 and 28.2 Kg/m^2 from the groups 1–5, respectively.

- The mean systolic blood pressure was 122.0 mmHg, 138.8 mmHg, 145.0 mmHg, 130.0 mmHg and 133.6 mmHg from groups 1 to 5, respectively, and diastolic blood pressure was 77.7 mmHg, 80.1 mmHg, 84.0 mmHg, 89.5 mmHg and 92.0 mmHg from the groups 1–5, respectively.

- Association and correlation of trace metals and semen quality shows that calcium, magnesium, zinc, copper and selenium shows a positive correlation, whereas the sodium, potassium, chromium, and lead shows the negative correlation with semen parameters.

- The mean calcium concentration in seminal plasma was observed as 10.6 mg/dL, 15.5 mg/dL and 18.6 mg/dL in groups 1 to 3, respectively but the groups 4 and 5 show slightly higher concentration (22.6 mg/dL and 24.2 mg/dL).

- The mean magnesium concentration in semen plasma of the study participants and it was noticed that 2.2 mEq/L (group 1); 2.9 mEq/L (group 2); 5.4 mEq/L (group 3); 4.3 mEq/L (group 4) and 8.5 mEq/L (group 5) respectively.

- The mean zinc level was 6.3 mg/dL, 4.1 mg/dL, 2.0 mg/dL, 1.6 mg/dL, and 1.4 mg/dL in groups, 1–5 respectively.

- The mean Na level was 148.3 mEq/L, 139.4 mEq/L, 132.0 mEq/L, 128.8 mEq/L and 120.2 mEq/L in groups 1–5, respectively.

- The mean K level was 5.0 mEq/L, 13.2 mEq/L, 22.8 mEq/L, 22.4 mEq/L and 22.6 mEq/L.

- The mean copper concentration was 81.0 μg/dL, 142.0 μg/dL, 154.0 μg/dL, 149.0 μg/dL and 167.0 μg/dL in groups 1–5, respectively.

- The selenium concentration was 178.2 μg/L (group 1), 77.6 μg/L (group 2), 52.2 μg/L (group 3), 56.4 μg/L (group 4) and 47.3 μg/L (group 5) respectively.

- Chromium concentration was assessed on seminal plasma and the results show that 2.2 μg/L, 4.2 μg/L, 4.9 μg/L, 4.6 μg/L and 5.8 μg/L in groups 1–5, respectively.

- The mean lead concentration in seminal plasma was 19.34 µg/L, 40.24 µg/L, 156.34 µg/L, 161.24 µg/L and 175.4 µg/L in groups 1–5, respectively.
- Pearson correlation was applied to study the association between the hormone level and semen parameters of the study groups and the results show that TSH, FSH, LH and PRL shows a negative correlation but TST level shows a positive correlation with semen parameters.
- The mean TSH was 2.5 µIU/mL, 2.2 µIU/mL, 6.5 µIU/mL, 7.4 µIU/mL and 10.0 µIU/mL in groups 1–5, respectively.
- The mean FSH was 5.1 mIU/mL (group 1), 4.9 mIU/mL (group 2), 12.1 mIU/mL (group 3), 14.6 mIU/mL (group 4) and 16.8 mIU/mL (group 5) respectively.
- The mean LH level was 4.6 mIU/mL, 4.5 mIU/mL, 8.6 mIU/mL, 10.0 mIU/mL and 12.3 mIU/mL in groups 1–5, respectively.
- The mean PRL was 10.3 ng/mL in group 1, 12.2 ng/mL in group 2, 14.9 ng/mL in group 3, 20.4 ng/mL in group 4 and 25.4 ng/mL in group 5.
- The mean TST level was 840.1 ng/dL in group 629.9 ng/dL in group 440.3 ng/dL in group 412.5 ng/dL in group 4 and 338.8 ng/dL in group 5 respectively.
- Association of semen quality parameters with behavior measures of the study participants shows that occupation, fertility duration, stress, tight underwear, diet, smoking and alcohol consumption shows a negative correlation.
- The mean sperm count was higher in IT group (38.3 million/mL) and lower (36.6 million/mL) other industries group. Mean sperm motility was observed as 30.2% and 28.9% in IT and other industries respectively. Higher normal morphology was found in IT (5.2%) and compared to other industries (5.0%).
- The mean sperm count was highest in fertility duration <5 years group (43.6 million/mL) and lower in fertility duration >5 years group (36.6 million/mL). Mean sperm motility was observed at 32.7% and 29.9% in fertility duration <5 years and >5 years respectively. Higher normal morphology was found in fertility duration <5 years (6.2%) and compared to >5 years (6.0%).

- The mean sperm count (62.0 million/mL) was observed maximum in the low stress group compared to high stress (31.9 million/mL). Similarly the mean sperm motility was 38.1% in low stress and 28.4% in the high stress group. The mean sperm morphology was found maximum (8.2%) in low stress compared to high stress (5.1%) group.

- The mean sperm count (34.0 million/mL) was lower in tight underwear group compare to normal (41.5 million/mL). The mean sperm motility (30.7%) was observed higher in normal compared to tight underwear group (25.0%). Similarly the mean morphology (3.6%) was lower in tight underwear group compared to normal (5.9%). Low sperm count (43.7 million/mL), motility (36.9%), morphology (7.0%) was observed in non-vegetarians compared to vegetarians (count: 44.1 million/mL, motility: 39.1% and morphology: 7.5%).

- The low sperm count (36.5 million/mL), motility (26.8%) and morphology (4.5%) was observed in smokers compared to non-smoker (count: 47.9 million/mL, motility: 38.5% and morphology (8.6%) and the low sperm count (36.1 million/mL), motility (28.5%) and morphology (5.3%) was observed in alcoholic compared to non-alcoholic participants (count: 55.8 million/mL, motility: 40.9% and morphology (8.8%).

- It was found that the vitamin D concentration in seminal plasma was observed as 72.1 ng/mL, 23.8 ng/mL, 20.4 ng/dl, 13.3 ng/mL and 18.0 ng/mL in groups 1–5, respectively, and the mean sperm count ($r = 0.19$, $p<0.05$), sperm motility ($r = 0.09$, $p>0.05$) and morphology ($r = 0.19$; $p<0.05$), shows significant positive correlation with vitamin D level.

- It was observed that the DNA fragmentation was found high (15.2%) in the older age group (41–50 years) compare to younger age group (20–30 years) and higher DNA fragmentation was observed high (15.5%) in obese or overweight compare to norm BMI (11.6%) participants.

- The maximum (15.2%) DNA fragmentation was found in smokers compared to non-smokers (12.6%) and the 15.0% of DNA fragmentation was observed in alcoholics compared to non-alcoholics (13.4%).

6.0 CONCLUSION

This study concludes that there could be multiple factors that bring changes in semen quality among the study groups 2–5 when compared to group1. It was noticed that most of the semen parameters were not in normal range among groups 2–5.

It can be concluded from the results of this study that Ca, Mg, Zn, Cu, Se are essential elements for sperm count, motility and morphology, whereas the Na, K, Cr and Pb shows the negative correlation with semen parameters. It is essential to maintain normal limits in both blood and semen to ensure the routine fertility capacity of a man, but higher concentration proved to be toxic.

This study concludes that the hormone profiles play an important role in male infertility. It was observed that abnormal hormone levels in groups 2–5, which are significantly shows negative correlation with semen parameters when compared to the normal group. Pearson correlation shows that except testosterone and other hormones show a negative correlation with sperm count, motility and morphology.

From this study it was concluded that vitamin D was positively correlated with semen parameters include sperm count, motility and morphology. Higher and lower concentration of vitamin D influences the semen quality in abnormal groups compared to normal group.

This study concludes that sperm DNA damage is higher in the abnormal group compared to the normal group. It was further concluded that sperm DNA damage was gradually increasing along with age and BMI. The sperm DNA damage was specifically increased in subjects with smokers and alcohol consumer. For the confirmatory results, need further investigation with a larger sample size and also need a very detailed investigation of the study participants. However, more number of studies with adequate sample size may reveal additional information on the influence of all forms on seminal parameters.

CPSIA information can be obtained
at www.ICGtesting.com
Printed in the USA
LVHW040909060423
743581LV00010B/289

9 781805 250623